Praises for The
Healthy Lifestyle

These are just a few of the th[...]
we receive yearly, praising The Bra[...]
the rejuvenation benefits they reap – physically, mentally,
and spiritually. We look forward to hearing from you also.

When I was a young Stanford University gymnastic coach,
Paul Bragg's wise words and his example inspired me to
live a healthy lifestyle. I was twenty-three then; now I am
over sixty, and my health and fitness serves as a living
testimonial to Paul Bragg's wisdom, carried on by his health
crusading daughter, Dr. Patricia Bragg. Thank you!
– Dan Millman, Author, Way of the Peaceful Warrior
www.danmillman.com

What a wonderful difference I have felt physically,
mentally and, most important to me, spiritually.
– Tully Strong, Coos Bay, Oregon

The Bragg Healthy Lifestyle along with Fasting has changed
my life! I lost weight and my energy levels went through
the roof. I look forwared to "Fasting" days. I think better
and am a better husband and father. Thank you Patricia,
this has been a great blessing in my life. Also, we enjoyed
your sharing your health message at our "AOL" Conference.
– Byron H. Elton, VP Entertainment, Time Warner AOL

Thank you Paul and Patricia Bragg for my simple, easy
to follow Health Program. You make my days healthy!
– Clint Eastwood, Bragg follower for 49 years

Bragg Books were my conversion to the healthy way.
– James F. Balch, M.D.,
Co-Author "Prescription for Nutritional Healing"

Praises for The Bragg Health Teachings

Paul Bragg saved my life at age 15 when I attended the Bragg Health Crusade in Oakland. I thank the Bragg Healthy Lifestyle for my long, active, happy life spreading health.
– Jack LaLanne, Bragg follower for over 75 years

I've experienced a beautiful, remarkable, spiritual awakening since reading this book. I'll never be quite the same again.
– Sandy Tuttle, Painesville, Ohio

Your book gives me so much motivation when I need it. Thank you again for your inspiration, I am honored to be among your millions of health students worldwide.
– John F. Crann, Livingston, New Jersey

I am thrilled by what I've read in the Bragg Health Books. Thank you, I am confident of my new ways to health.
– Ken Cooper, D.C., Narrabi, NSW, Australia

I found your Bragg Vinegar book in a health store. I bought it, read it, gave copies to several friends, even including my doctor. I have followed The Bragg Healthy Lifestyle since. I can honestly say that out of all the books I have read, the Bragg Health Books have benefited me the most.
– Reiner Rothe, Vancouver, Canada

I am eternally grateful for your health books. They have made a great difference in my life. I'm sharing them with my friends.
– Carolyn Orfel, Washinton, D.C.

I am a Champion Weight Lifter at Muscle Beach for over 50 years and we are all big Bragg fans.
– Chris Baioa, Santa Monica, California

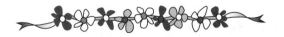

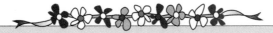

Praises for The Bragg Health Teachings

I would like to personally thank you for teaching me how to take control of my health! I have lost almost 55 pounds. I feel "Great". These books have shown me happiness, vitality and living close to Mother Nature and God. You are a super person, a real crusader of "Health". – Leonard Amato

---

Thank you – My family and I are faithfully following your Bragg Healthy Lifestyle and enjoying the great benefits.
– Dr. Jan Buscop, South Africa

I have faithfully followed your Healthy Lifestyle and I now use your Bragg Liquid Aminos not only for my own food but in dilution for my plants. – Daley Machado, Brazil

---

You have recharged me with hope, encouragement and love which poured from your words. I'm now able to fast and no more cigarettes and coffee for me, you've certainly improved my life! – Marie Furia, West Orange, New Jersey

---

I have utilized your book's precepts and in turn have reaped overflowing health, joy and energy.
– Gill Contreras, Texarkana, Texas

I have lost all my excess weight with fasting and following your teachings. Now my friends are starting to live the Bragg healthy way too. – R. Cortez, Upland, California

---

Your fasting book has renewed my youth. I'm 58 years young and feel 18, and I can outrun 18 year olds! Through your fasting plan, I lost over 86 pounds and feel a sense of rejuvenated youthfulness.
– Donald Daigh, Key West, Flordia

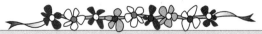

Praises for The Bragg Health Teachings

How did I beat cancer, obesity, diabetes, strep, three herniated disks and excruciating pain? The answer was changing to the Bragg's Healthy Lifestyle Program! It changed and saved my life! I had full recovery and also lost over 70 lbs. I received a new life and that is just the beginning because my manhood returned that was lost to diabetes – now that's exciting. On my trip to Honolulu, Hawaii I visited the famous free Bragg Exercise Class at Waikiki Beach. I became so regenerated with a wonderful new viewpoint towards living my healthy lifestyle that I now live in Hawaii. I'm invigorated with new energy. My new purpose for living is to help others reclaim their health rights! I also want the world to join The Bragg Health Crusade. I am deeply thankful to Health Crusaders Paul and Patricia Bragg for my new healthy life!

– Len Schneider, Honolulu, Hawaii

I'm keeping healthy and fit and love Bragg Liquid Amino Seasoning. My mother uses Braggs in most of her recipes.

– Mary Pierce, French Tennis Champion

Paul and Patricia Bragg were my early inspiration to my health education. – Jeffery Bland, Ph.D, Food Scientist

---

We get letters daily at our Santa Barbara headquarters. We would love to receive a testimonial from you on any blessings, healings and changes you experienced after following The Bragg Healthy Lifestyle and our Fasting detox program. It's all within your grasp to be in top health. By following this book, you can reap Super Health and a happy, long, vital life! It's never too late to begin. Read the study (page 49) they did with people in their 80s and 90s and the amazing results that were obtained. Receive miracles with natural nutrition, exercise and fasting! Start now!

To the readers of Bragg Health Books. . .
Daily our prayers & love go out to you, your heart, mind & soul.

3 John 2   *Patricia Bragg*   Genesis 6:3

D

Miracles can happen every day through guidance and prayer! – Patricia Bragg

BRAGG

BUILD STRONG HEALTHY FEET

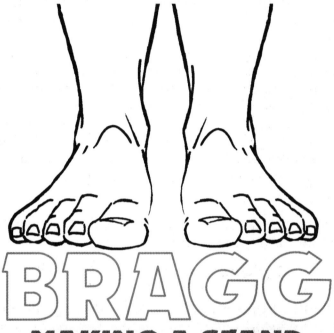

MAKING A STAND
For HEALTHY FEET

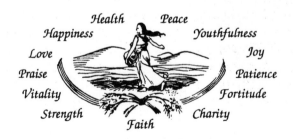

Health   Peace
Happiness   Youthfulness
Love   Joy
Praise   Patience
Vitality   Fortitude
Strength   Charity
Faith

BECOME

A Bragg Health Crusader – for a 100% Healthy World for All!

HEALTH SCIENCE

Box 7, Santa Barbara, California 93102 USA

World Wide Web: www.bragg.com

Notice: Our writings are to help guide you to live a healthy lifestyle and prevent health problems. If you suspect you have a medical problem, please seek alternative health professionals to help you make the healthiest informed choices. Diabetics should fast only under a health professional's supervision! If hypoglycemic, add Spirulina or barley green powder to liquids when fasting.

BRAGG

BUILD
STRONG
HEALTHY
FEET

PAUL C. BRAGG, N.D., Ph.D.
LIFE EXTENSION SPECIALIST
and
PATRICIA BRAGG, N.D., Ph.D.
HEALTH & FITNESS EXPERT

Health Science, Box 7, Santa Barbara, California 93102
Telephone (805) 968-1020, FAX (805) 968-1001
e-mail address: books@bragg.com

Quantity Purchases: Companies, Professional Groups, Churches, Clubs, Fundraisers, etc. Please contact our Special Sales Department.

**To see Bragg Books and Products on-line,
visit our Website at: www.bragg.com**

This book is printed on recycled, acid-free paper.

- REVISED AND EXPANDED -
Copyright © Health Science
Fifteenth Printing MMIV
ISBN: 0-87790-056-6

Published in the United States
HEALTH SCIENCE, Box 7, Santa Barbara, California 93102 USA

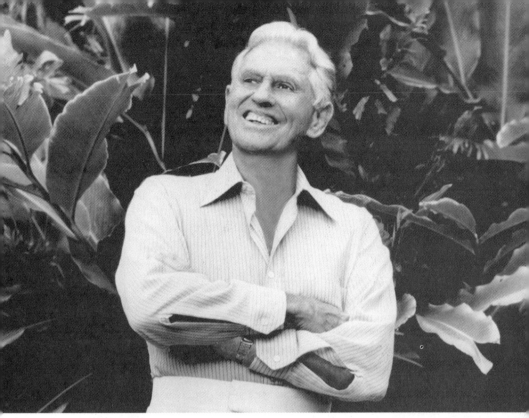

PAUL C. BRAGG, N.D., Ph.D.
World's Leading Healthy Lifestyle Authority

Paul C. Bragg's daughter Patricia and their wonderful, healthy members of the Bragg *Longer Life, Health and Happiness Club* exercise daily on the beautiful Fort DeRussy lawn, at famous Waikiki Beach in Honolulu, Hawaii. *View the club exercising:* www.bragg.com. Membership is free and open to everyone to attend any morning – Monday through Saturday, from 9 to 10:30 am – for Bragg Super Power Breathing and Health and Fitness Exercises. On Saturday there are often health lectures on how to live a long, healthy life! The group averages 75 to 125 per day, depending on the season. From December to March it can go up to 150. Its dedicated leaders have been carrying on the class for over 30 years. Thousands have visited the club from around the world and carried the Bragg Health and Fitness Crusade to friends and relatives back home. When you visit Honolulu, Hawaii, Patricia invites you and your friends to join her and the club for wholesome, healthy fellowship. She also recommends visiting the outer Islands (Kauai, Hawaii, Maui, Molokai) for a fulfilling, healthy vacation.

To maintain good health, normal weight and increase the good life of radiant health, joy and happiness, the body must be exercised properly (stretching, walking, jogging, running, biking, swimming, deep breathing, good posture, etc.) and nourished wisely with healthy foods. – Paul C. Bragg

BRAGG HEALTH CRUSADES for 21st Century
Teaching People Worldwide to Live Healthy, Happy, Stronger, Longer Lives for a Better World

We love sharing and teaching healthy living world-wide, and you can share this love by being a partner by sharing The Bragg Health Crusades message. We are dedicated with a passion to help others! We feel blessed when you and your family's lives improve through following our teachings from the Bragg Health Books and The Bragg Health Crusades. It makes our years of faithful service so worthwhile! We will keep sharing, and please do write us how our teachings have helped you.

The Miracle of Fasting book has been the #1 Health book for over 20 years in Russia, the Ukraine and now in Bulgaria! Why? Because we show them how to live a healthy, wholesome life for less money, and it's so easy to understand and follow. Most healthful lifestyle habits are free (good posture, clean thoughts, plain natural food, exercise and deep breathing, all of which promotes energy and health into the body). We continue to reach the multitudes worldwide with our health books and teachings, lectures, crusades, radio and TV outreaches.

My joy and priorities come from God, Mother Nature and healthy living. I love being a health crusader and spreading health worldwide, for now it's needed more than ever! My father and I also pioneered Health TV with our program "Health and Happiness" from Hollywood. Yes – it's thrilling to be a Health Crusader and you will enjoy it also. See back pages to list names (yourself, family and friends) who you feel would benefit from receiving our free Health Bulletins!

By reading Bragg Self-Health Books you gain a new confidence that you can help yourself, family and friends to The Bragg Healthy Principles of Living! Please call your local book stores and health stores and ask for the Bragg Health Books. Prayerfully, we hope to have all stores stock the books. We do keep prices as low as possible, so they will be affordable and available for everyone to learn how to live and enjoy a healthier, happier and longer life!

With Blessings of Health, Peace and Love,

Patricia Bragg

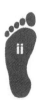

BRAGG HEALTH CRUSADES, America's Health Pioneers
Keep Bragg Health Crusades "Crusading" with your tax deductible donations.
Box 7, Santa Barbara, CA 93102 USA (805) 968-1020
Spreading health worldwide since 1912

ii

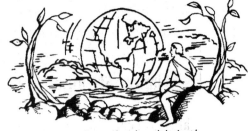

BRAGG BUILD STRONG HEALTHY FEET

To preserve health is a moral and religious duty, for health is the basis for all social virtues. We can no longer be as useful when not well.
– Dr. Samuel Johnson, Father of Dictionaries

Contents

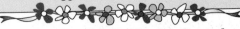

Bragg Healthy Lifestyle Plan

- Read, plan, plot, and follow through for supreme health and longevity.
- Underline, highlight or dog-ear pages as you read important passages.
- Organizing your lifestyle helps you identify what's important in your life.
- Be faithful to your health goals everyday for a healthy, strong, happy life.
- Write us about your successes following The Bragg Healthy Lifestyle.
- Where space allows we have included "words of wisdom" from great minds to motivate and inspire you. Please share some of your favorites with us.

The Bragg Books are written to inspire and guide you to radiant health and longevity. Remember, the book you don't read won't help. Please reread our Books often and live The Bragg Healthy Lifestyle for a long, happy, fulfilled life!

Remember – your feet are miracles in motion – be good to them!
– Paul C. Bragg, Health Crusader, and Originator of Health Stores

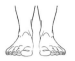

Contents

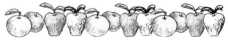

What you are is God's gift to you.
What you make of yourself is your gift to God.

Contents

Make your two feet your best friends. – J. M. Barrie

The natural healing force within us is the greatest force in getting well.
– Hippocrates, Father of Medicine, 400 BC

Friendship is to people, what sunshine is to flowers

v

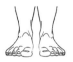

Contents

*People who maintain a healthy ideal, trim body weight can lower
their risk of heart disease as much as 55%.* – American Heart Association

Contents

*Bragg Books are silent health teachers – never tiring,
ready night or day to help you help yourself to health!*

Learning and Growth promote happiness! – Pearl S. Buck

Helpful Exercise Tips to Make Air Travel More Healthy and Comfortable:

• Contact airlines special service department and arrange seating on aisle for more leg room, or bulkhead seat for more leg room and comfort.
• Exercises keep your muscles working and prevent back spasms.
• Sit and stretch up spine, now, turn your head to the right, then hold for ten seconds and bring back to the front, then repeat excercise to left. Do 5 sets.
• Keep arms by sides and do this shoulder roll: shrug shoulders upward to ears, now roll shoulders back, down and around. Do 5 sets each way.
• Shoes off are best – Lift heels so balls of feet are still on floor, then drop heels back to floor, now stretch toes up and rotate feet around. Do 10 sets each way.
• Walk along aisles and in corridors. Do back arches, by placing hands in small of back and gently arch backwards. Also, do side bends by placing hands on hips and bend gently to right, hold five seconds, and back to upright, then bend to left. Do 10 sets. (See Web: *www.backcare.com*)

Exercising in the Sky – You Arrive Healthier

We even jog while thousands of feet high in the air, soaring the skies in an airplane. We go to rear of the plane and stationary jog and stretch. This gives your billions of cells a massage. We never arrive stiff and tired. Also learn to take advantage of spare moments for a stationary jog daily, whether an office worker, CEO or housewife. We all need to exercise for healthy bones, a strong heart and a healthy body! Millions are traveling by air, but for people with back pain, air travel can be painful and difficult. Narrow seat widths and more seats being added to pack airplanes to capacity causes air passengers to have less leg room and a problem for those who suffer back and leg pain!

Remember to ask for a bulkhead or an exit row seat for more leg room.

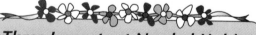

Three Important Needed Habits

There are three habits which, with one condition added, that will give you everything in the world worth having, beyond which the imagination of man cannot conjure forth a single additional improvement! These habits are:
• The Health Habit • The Work Habit • The Study Habit
If you have these habits, and also the love of God and someone who has these habits, you are both in paradise now and here. – Elbert Hubbard

When you sell a man a book you don't just sell him paper, ink and glue, you sell him a whole new life! There's heaven and earth in a real book. The real purpose of books is to trap the mind into its own thinking! – Christopher Morley

Love makes the world go 'round; it's everlasting when it's written with caring, loving advice that will improve and enrich your life! This is why my father and I love sharing with you our health wisdoms which can be with you on your long life's journey. Our books on health, fitness and longevity go around the world spreading health and love! – Patricia Bragg, N.D.,Ph.D.

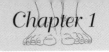

Chapter 1

Nature's Way to Healthy, Strong and Happy Feet

The Basics of Foot Functions

Almost all of us are born with perfect feet. It's the abuse millions give their feet that makes them limp into adulthood crying, *My aching feet are killing me!*

The foot is a complex, elegant and delicately balanced miracle mechanism. Perfect balance is essential to foot comfort, and the maintenance of this balance depends upon healthy natural foot function.

Almost all types of shoes made disturb the delicate balance of the feet, to the extent that they cannot endure the jars and missteps in addition to walking on the hard city streets which can upset the normal foot function. This results in either tension or locking of the joints, painful strain in the arches, muscles and limitation of foot motion or a combination of these disturbances. The direct consequence is discomfort: aches and pains in the feet, legs, knees, thighs and back!

As long as this amazing, balanced foot function is maintained, your feet will be comfortable. No matter how out of shape your feet may appear, if they can be made to function at least 85% normally, then pain disappears, miracles happen and soon with loving care your feet will look and feel healthy and youthful again!

Now, let us demonstrate what we mean by foot function or the coordination of its many intricate parts. Do this experiment now – before you read further – and you will understand at once the natural or unnatural (as this may be) function of the feet. Stand on one foot (without shoes) and without support, try to maintain your balance for a few minutes. If your foot function is normal, balance will be maintained with perfect ease.

1

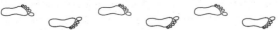

The foot, a work of art, is an engineering masterpiece! – Leonardo daVinci

Perfect Balance or No Balance

If foot function is impaired, balance will be difficult. You will tire in a short time and even sometimes in minutes can suffer leg pains. Observe what happens: at once the inner side of the foot comes into rapid play or action, with slight, constantly fluctuating adjustments necessary to sustain the body balance; the outer side of the foot remains comparatively immobile and your entire weight tends to focus upon that part.

The fluctuating inner part of the foot is called the *spring-arch*. Its chief function is to adjust for and maintain balance. The outer portion is called the *weight-bearing arch* and it operates to center and sustain the body weight.

By this simple experiment, you will learn not only the importance of the structure of your feet, but you will also be able to test their condition. The normal, unimpaired foot will balance the body perfectly, with graceful, easy movements and only a slight swaying of the body. The weak, crippled or deformed foot will make violent jerky efforts to balance the body, but will fail! Impaired function will force you to reach for support, to drop the other foot to the ground, or fall in a heap.

The condition of a great majority of feet are between the extremes of Perfect Balance and No Balance. The vital importance of this balancing action of the foot becomes evident the moment we consider the act of walking. While walking, we are continuously balancing first on one foot and then on the other as we transfer the weight of the body forward from right to left and left to right. In fact, it is a movement demanding remarkable equipoise, for the height and mass of the human body are out of proportion architecturally to the narrow base formed by the feet. The equilibrium, in turn, depends upon the perfect coordination of the nerves and muscles and their control of the lever-like bones, fulcrums, bases, angles and shifting surface of the feet. Correct walking is a feat of balancing on balanced feet!

It's supposed to be a professional secret, but I'll tell you anyway. We doctors do nothing. We only help and encourage the doctor within. – Albert Schweitzer

Since most all foot comfort depends upon normal foot function, beware of diagnosis of arthritis or so-called rheumatism when the lower extremities are painful, since nearly all these symptoms can stem from some functional foot disturbance to even overweight and poor posture. For more info., refer to the section on gout, arthritis and rheumatism in the *Senior Steps* section of Chapter Six.

Causes of Broken Arches

Nearly all foot troubles are the result of various injuries. The most common injury is caused by shoes that do not properly conform to the foot and hence, do not permit free and natural foot performance. Quite often, students are surprised when we tell them that their feet are not functioning normally. It is hard to make them understand that bones are actually dislocated. The reason this bone displacement occurs is simple and plausible. The feet, relative to their size, do more work than any other part of the body. They are subjected to injury every day. Wrong ill-fitting shoes, missteps, sprains, pounding on hard sidewalks, etc. all take their toll! The cumulative effect of all this punishment finally displaces the bones, upsets the balanced function and pain is the result. The body's *walking gear* is slowly being put out of adjustment!

Bad Walking Habits Bring Miseries

One of the early signs is the eversion, or outward turning of the foot. From here serious foot troubles start! We are walking out of natural foot and body balance. This affects all of the bones and nerves of the feet, and in turn the ankle, calf, knee and hip. This results in the knee being thrown out of balance, as well as thighs, etc. *The hip and lower spine are pushed out of alignment. The trouble travels up the spine, also resulting in misplacement of shoulders and head. Pains and miseries are felt throughout the body.* This may be expected, when the feet are out of balance.

Man is fully responsible for his habits and his choices. – Jean Paul Sartre

Prevention is always preferable to the cure.

Women have four times as many foot problems as men do.

3

Again, let us say, these pains will be given many names from arthritis to curvature of the spine or you may be told you have slipped discs of the vertebrae, etc. The basic cause of all your pain, however, may be that you are completely out of foot-balance, thus throwing your entire body out of line! If you have curvature of the spine, be sure to see our *Bragg Back Fitness Program* book. Please see the back pages of this book for the Bragg Booklist.

The actual mechanism in the foot, after it becomes everted, is disturbed by a specific displacement of certain bones in the arches. These bones become jammed into a position of extreme tension that strains the ligaments and also the arch muscles. The results are a marked impairment of foot action and a complete change in weight-bearing forces. Due to changes in equilibrium, the body is thrown forward so that the muscles have to compensate and thus work overtime to keep the body erect. The body muscles are straining, just as if a person were continually walking downhill and holding the body erect to compensate for the grade. This effect brings into unnatural play the legs, back and neck muscles, which can soon become tired and ache.

The fundamental abnormality, as it exists in the vast majority of cases, is a specific displacement of certain bones of the feet. This causes limited foot action and prolonged arch strain, these being two conditions which are usually responsible for disturbing foot pains.

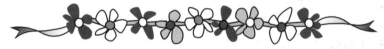

Laughter is inner jogging and good for your body and soul. – Norman Cousins

Dream big, think big, but enjoy the small miracles of everyday life!

Man's body was created according to the laws of physics and chemistry, which are the Creator's own laws. They never vary. His law is written upon every cell, every nerve, every muscle, every faculty, which has been entrusted to us to care for and protect. – Henry W. Vollmer, M.D.

4

Living under conditions of our modern life, it's important to bear in mind that the preparation and refinement of food products can either entirely eliminate or in part destroy the vital elements in the original food material. – U.S. Dept. of Agriculture, visit web: www.usda.gov

The Many Causes of Foot Problems

- Shoes that mold and push the feet out of alignment cause mounting trouble unless shoes conform to the foot.
- Usage of unnaturally ill-fitting shoes, causing slow displacement of bones which limits foot and arch function and causes corns, bunions and foot problems.
- Womens high heels, can cause a multitude of painful symptoms as a result of distorted foot functions, and also throws the body's posture and organs out of line.
- Deficiencies of proper nutrients and protein, which prevent the building of a normal healthy foot.
- Deficiencies of the minerals like calcium and other bone-making nutrients can prevent the building and maintaining of healthy, strong feet.
- Insufficient and incorrect foot exercise, can result in weak feet. Foot muscles can't get full exercise when bound in shoes all the time (*go barefoot more often*).
- Bones of the feet require exercise to function correctly.
- All shoes hamper the full exercise of the 26 foot bones, also the ligaments don't get the exercise they need!

Foot Distress Symptoms

As a result of displaced bones and abnormal function, and with possible nutritional deficiencies of vitamins, minerals and protein, one may expect to have some of or all of the following Foot Distress Symptoms:

- Feet that feel like they are killing you.
- Cold feet that lack circulation.
- Bunions and corns.
- Extremely tired feet and legs.
- Weak and sore arches.
- Aching and cramping muscles in feet and arches.
- Pain in heels, especially when walking and standing.
- Burning sensations; numbness.
- Aching, cramping leg muscles into ankle areas.
- Painful thighs, hips and back.
- Stiff and painful knees.
- Painful calluses at points of undue weight-bearing.
- Difficulty with balance on rough surfaces.
- Fatigue, headaches, irritability, nervous exhaustion.

Follow Mother Nature and God – the rewards are great! – Patricia Bragg

The Importance of Foot Education

We can now plainly see that most foot troubles are mainly caused by ill-fitting shoes, lack of exercise, poor posture and various vitamin and mineral deficiencies. That is the reason this foot care program was written, to help you regain the feeling of healthy, strong, youthful feet!

No matter how deformed the feet may appear, if the nutrition and function can be improved, the pains will be lessened and the feet will feel stronger! To the health student this is very welcome news. It means that he or she may get comfort, even while having the worst-looking feet. But it also means that a person is not necessarily immune from functional and nutritional foot disorders simply because he or she possesses perfect-looking feet. Even beautiful looking feet may give you problems, too. What we really want are healthy, strong, serviceable feet that you can use for hours upon hours without the slightest sign of pain or fatigue! This is what we will strive for you in this Foot Care Program. No matter how much trouble you are experiencing with your feet, you are now going to treat them as Mother Nature intended you to and improvement will begin!!!

Major Foot Bones

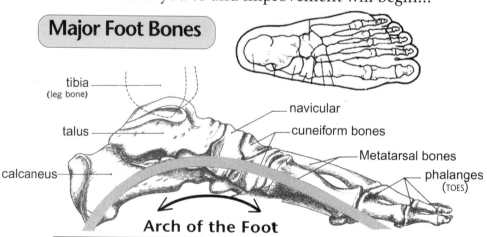

tibia (leg bone)

talus

calcaneus

navicular

cuneiform bones

Metatarsal bones

phalanges (TOES)

Arch of the Foot

Treatment of the feet to improve comfort and function will favorably affect other parts of the body. – Elizabeth H. Roberts, D.P.M.

Sad-many people go through life committing partial slow suicide destroying their health, feet, youth, beauty, talents, energies and creative qualities. Indeed, to learn how to be good to oneself is often more difficult than to learn how to be good to others. – Paul C. Bragg

6

25% of the body's bones are in the feet.

Go Barefoot for Healthy, Youthful Feet!

The first step in building healthy, new feet is to go barefoot at every opportunity, and please stop worrying about catching a cold when going barefoot (Diabetics only go barefoot at home and it's best they wear socks). You don't catch colds from walking on cold floors or other surfaces. This old rumor should have been discarded hundreds of years ago! Colds are Mother Nature's way of purging the body of toxic poisons. They are the safety valve that lets the poisons leave the body. A cold is God's blessing to you! Think of all the body waste, mucus and poison released from your bloodstream, nose, lungs, etc. when you have a cold. Remember that the body has its own repair shop built right into it. Your miracle body when given the opportunity, is self-cleansing, self-repairing and healing!

Whenever you can get your shoes off (home, car, office, etc.), please do so! Most shoes, clogs, sandals and foot covers of all kinds can impede natural foot function. It's usually the combination of poor nutrition and improperly fitted shoes that cause most foot troubles, directly or indirectly.

India-China Foot Survey Proves Barefoot Best!

Perhaps nothing can illustrate the foregoing more graphically than a foot survey taken years ago in India and China among people who habitually go barefoot. In the United States, similar foot surveys and studies revealed that about 85% of the adult population is foot defective, whereas the India-China Survey of some 5,000 people showed only a low 7% incidence of foot defects! Please do take care of your foot health and protect your feet and total well-being! Never neglect your feet and health and become a burden to yourself and perhaps to your family and others! See web: *www.barefooters.org*

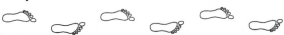

Shoes were unknown to our ancient forefathers; they went barefoot! But we squeeze our feet into shoes, losing direct contact with the ground. It's a central problem. It may sound trivial, but by wearing shoes we deprive our organs of the benefits provided by the reflex zones on our feet. What's even worse, the lack of ventilation and the constant pressure (caused by "fashionable" footwear that's often much too tight and small) causes calluses, corns, hammertoes, and other deformities. – Jurgen Jora, Foot Reflexology Visual Guide For Self-Treatment.

Written in the Pacific Paradise of Hawaii

We are writing this Bragg Foot Care Health Program at our home in Hawaii. The Hawaiian beach boys and girls, who seldom wear shoes, have perfect feet. Here in Hawaii, so many people go barefoot or wear just a light sandal that gives most Hawaiian's feet more freedom. As a result of going barefoot, these wonderful people of the Hawaiian Islands have the healthiest, happiest feet in the world. Almost everyone does the native Hula dance, which is never done in shoes or sandals of any kind!

We know exactly what remark you are going to give us regarding this statement, "We cannot live in Hawaii and go barefoot and do the Hula dance." We thoroughly agree with you! But, we can learn a lesson from these happy people and go barefoot in our own homes and around our front and back yards. Even your local park lawn can be inviting! When we do wear shoes, they should be of the type that give the bones and muscles of the feet as much freedom as they need. When you are barefoot, the feet function as Mother Nature intended.

Sick Feet Mar Beauty and Health

From this day forward, make it a practice to spend as much time as possible going barefoot. Let your feet live the Natural Way! Next to the heart, the feet carry the greatest work load of any body part. Keep this in mind when you backslide on your Bragg Foot Care Program!

Tired, aching feet and wearing badly-fitted shoes can make your face tense and your expression unhappy and contribute to backaches, bad posture and many other ills. What's more, you tend to drag such feet, and that ungraceful habit alone can make you feel and look years older than you are! Occasionally you may have a foot problem serious enough to require medical attention, but generally you can keep your feet in top shape all by yourself! It's not difficult to do and worth all the effort.

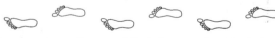

Researchers have discovered that the more healthy habits an individual practices, the longer they live and the healthier they are!
– Elizabeth Vierck, *Health Smart*

Toxic Acid Crystals Cement Joints

Toxic acid crystals can cement movable joints in your feet and make them stiff and fill them with misery and torment! Stand on any busy street corner and watch the people hobble along. Their feet, knees, hips, spine and head seem to be cemented, there is no free-swinging movement in their locomotion. Look at their feet. They seem to pick up their feet heavily and lay them down flatly. Their knees seem to be completely cemented and stiff. There is little movement or swinging motion in the hips. Their spines are rigid and so are their heads. All of the elasticity and resiliency seems to have gone out of what should be a smooth, free-swinging body.

Between the movable joints of every bone in the human body, Mother Nature at one time placed an abundant supply of lubrication known as synovial fluid. Take a look at a youngster who is 10 years of age and see the easy movement of every movable joint in the body. What is the reason that at 66 years old we can't have the freedom of motion in our joints that a child of 10 has? There is no reason! Years have nothing to do with the amount of synovial fluid that makes the joints move freely and easily. There is one main thing that cements your movable joints and that is toxic acid crystals!

Age is not toxic. Just because you live to be 60, 70, 80 or 90, there should be no diminishing of the supply of synovial fluid from age! Mother Nature does not stiffen and cement the joints of one person and not another; it is caused by the accumulation of toxins and acid crystals.

DEPOSITS OF INORGANIC MINERALS AND TOXIC ACID CRYSTALS CAUSE PAINFUL FEET!

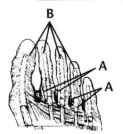

A. Deposited under tendons
B. Under the Achilles tendon
C. Under the heel
D. Under the middle foot

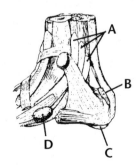

Inorganic mineral deposits that deposit themselves between the bones of the toes (**A** and **B**).

Poor Nutrition Causes Obesity & Toxic Buildup

By natural instinct, we eat when hungry, drink when thirsty and breathe air by necessity. Most humans eat way too much food mostly out of habit, not hunger! They have been brainwashed to believe you must have meals by the clock. They don't drink enough water. Thirst mimics their hunger and then they reach for the unhealthy snacks. We know from long experience that overweight people can't burn up these so-called regular meals. They are conditioned to eat breakfast whether they have a real hunger or not, so they load in ham, bacon, sausages, eggs, hot cakes, sweet rolls, doughnuts, toast, jelly, fried potatoes, waffles, coffee, sugar drinks, refined cereals and other body-wrecking junk foods.

Over 60% Americans are Overweight

The body does not have enough vital *Nerve Force* to masticate, digest, assimilate and eliminate these heavy breakfasts. There's always toxic residue left; and where does toxic residue go? It's concentrated and crystallized and finds its way into movable body joints. It's a slow unaware process until joints start to give trouble. It takes years of wrong eating to bring about heavy concentration to cause this acid crystal buildup in the movable joints.

When these calcium-like spurs attach themselves on the joints and calcified substances replace the synovial fluid, then pains and aches are felt in the body's movable joints. The first place they attack is usually the feet. Each foot has 26 movable bones, more than in any part of the body. Gravity sends the toxic crystals to the feet. Gradually the feet and the ankles start to stiffen because the toxic acid crystals replace the lubrication in the foot joints. So instead of the feet staying healthy and flexible, they gradually harden and cement. From the feet and ankles, as time marches on, the toxic acid crystals move up, causing many people to suffer from knee and hip pains from joint deterioration. When toxic crystals have moved into the hip joints, you can see by the way people move their hips that they are stiff and painful! Start observing peoples' walk and posture.

How to Flush Out Hardened Acid Crystals

Remember that acid crystals have been building up in your feet from the toxic and dead foods you have eaten all your life. It has taken a long time for you to build up these acid crystals. Some people not only build acid crystals but, they also build acid spurs on their foot bones, and these can cause excruciating pain. Sometimes sharp crystals bring on such intense pain because it's no longer possible for the body to break them down. At this point surgery is sometimes the only way to remove spurs that have attached themselves to the movable foot joints. In ordinary cases, toxic acid crystals can be removed by the person themselves with a careful hygienic foot plan, as in this book. This includes a health hygiene with foot therapy, water treatment, massage, reflexology, exercise, natural nutrition and fasting.

Fasting is one of the quickest ways to dissolve the acid crystals or spurs from the feet *(fasting also normalizes weight & blood pressure)*, but don't expect miracles to happen overnight. These crystals have taken many years to accumulate and sometimes it will take many dedicated months to dissolve them. The first thing to do is to complete a 24-hour water-only fast weekly. Then, occasionally take longer fasts. Our book, *The Miracle of Fasting* (page 28), covers the hows and whys of fasting in much greater detail than we could go into here. Other Bragg Health Books that will help you on your quest for perfectly functioning feet are: • *Water – The Shocking Truth That Can Save Your Life* • *Bragg Apple Cider Vinegar Miracle Health System*. See back pages for Bragg Booklist.

Remember, too much meat in the diet can result in a buildup of acid spurs in the feet. Meat contains a powerful toxin known as uric acid and the heavy meat eater will often suffer from acid crystals in their feet. Eggs, cheese and all dairy products are basically on the acidic side, so there must be caution in eating animal products of any kind!

Everything in excess is opposed by nature. – Hippocrates

It's a lean horse for the long, successful race of life!

Gravity and air pressure play an important part in the depositing of acid crystals in the feet. Remember, we live in an ocean of oxygen which reaches 70 miles high and weighs 14 pounds per square inch. This pressure constantly drives the toxic acid crystals to our lower extremities: the feet, ankles and knees. You only have to watch passing crowds on the street to see stiffness in the movable joints of the feet, knees, hips and lower back. What people call age is not due to passing of time, what we call chronological time; it is due to the accumulation and retention of toxic poisons that we take in when we eat unhealthy meals and live an unhealthy lifestyle!

Chronological or Biological Age?

So many humans want to blame the passage of time for the deterioration in their physical body. If you ask a foot sufferer over 50 what causes his stiffness, aches and pains, he will answer, "When you get older you get stiff." This is not true! Age is not toxic; the ticking of the clock, the passing of days, weeks, months and years can have no material effect upon the feet if the diet has a great preponderance of organic fruits and vegetables, raw or properly cooked. Most people do not follow natural and scientific nutrition. When painful toxic acid crystals build up in their feet and other parts of the body, most people erroneously want to blame it on their age.

Here's an illustration of what we are talking about. Chronologically, a person can be 80 years old, but biologically, they can be half that age. This is because that person slowed down the clock of time by adopting and following a strict program of natural living: correct exercises, deep breathing, healthy eating and drinking habits, plus detox fasting and other hygienic measures.

Relieved of the work of digesting foods, fasting permits the body to rid itself of toxins while facilitating healing. Fasting regularly gives your organs a rest and helps reverse the ageing process for a longer and healthier life.
– James Balch, M.D., Prescription for Nutritional Healing
"Bragg Books were my conversion to the healthy way."

Elimination of body toxins and waste by fasting increases longevity.
– Alexis Carrel, M.D., famous scientist, Rockefeller Institute
see web: nobel.sdsc.edu/medicine/laureates/1912/carrel-bio.html

Once, while we were at a social gathering, a man on crutches complained to us that his feet were so painful he had to ease the pressure with crutches as he walked. His feet were in a horrible condition. They were so full of the accumulated acid crystals and toxic waste, he even had to wear oversized slippers. Not only did he suffer from bad feet, but he also had protruding varicose veins (pooled blood) on the right leg and two open running varicose ulcers. Now this is not all that was wrong with the gentleman. He told us that he had hardening of the arteries, an irregular heartbeat (arrythmia), cataracts on both of his eyes and he had lost the ability to hear well. This man was only 62 chronological years old. Again, we want to emphasize to you that your bad feet are not due to your age, but to the way you have lived!

Here is your program for rejuvenating your feet, for putting back vitality, energy and the spring in your step that belongs to them! Study this program seriously. Take the time to take care of your feet, then they will work hard and faithfully for you if you will give them the care and attention that they need!

It's Important to Bathe Your Feet Properly

Don't scoff at the suggestion that you may not know how to bathe your feet properly. Like so many other simple facts about health care, this is one you are apt to take for granted, which can lead to trouble! There's more to bathing your feet than just casually dabbing them with soap when you take your bath. With your daily bath or shower it is important to pay more attention to foot cleansing and foot therapy! (See pages 15-17.)

The human body has one ability not possessed by any machine, the ability to repair and heal itself. – George E. Crile, Jr. M.D.

During the average American's lifetime, their feet will carry them the equivalent of 5 times around the earth! – www.apma.org

---

Shocking Facts: *America's tragic nationwide health care costs soared to $900 billion back in 1993 and is expected to more than double by 2005. This is all the more reason each American should live The Bragg Healthy Lifestyle to save our economy from this huge medical expense, not to mention the premature death and suffering (physical, mental, emotional and financial).*

13

Nature's Antiseptic – Tea Tree Oil

Oil derived from the Tea Tree leaves can be used for treating skin abrasions, acne, canker sores and foot fungus, says William J. Keller Ph.D., herbal expert and chair of the department of Pharmaceutical Sciences at Samford University McWhorter School of Pharmacy (www.samford.edu). The Tea Tree (melaleuca alternifolia) is a member of the Myrtaceae family and is indigenous to New South Wales, Australia. It was used as a general antiseptic by aboriginal tribes for thousands of years. The name is credited to Captain Cook, who in 1770, brewed the leaves for his men to prevent scurvy. In 1923 clinical trials in Australia provided strong scientific evidence of Tea Tree Oil's antiseptic and bactericidal properties and its importance made it a standard issue for the Australian Army during World War II.

Here are more tips from Doctor Keller on Treating Athlete's Foot and Black Toenails using Tea Tree Oil:

• Start applying Tea Tree Oil lightly right from bottle. Full strength may over-dry skin. If skin becomes flaky, then dilute oil by mixing 3 Tea Tree Oil with q Bragg Organic Virgin Olive Oil or Jojoba Oil, or mix all 3 oils.

• Apply Tea Tree Oil to area 3 times a day. Continue treatment for one week after infection disappears.

• A few people might be allergic to Tea Tree Oil, so use a very small dab the first time to check if you are.

For smelly feet, nightly you can enjoy a Tea Tree Oil foot soak (add 5 to 10 drops to warm water in shallow pan). Great while reading or watching TV, continue until improvement. Use oil along with Tea Tree Foot Powder or Tea Tree Foot Spray, available health stores. For more Athlete's Foot info see pages 15,18,79,80,108,111,112,115,137. For more Tea Tree info see this website : *www.teatree.co.uk*

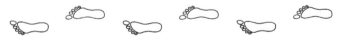

Sad Facts: Around 80% of adult Americans have foot problems at some time in their life.
– American Orthopedic Foot and Ankle Society, www.aofas.org

Now learn what and how great benefits a temperate diet will bring with it. In the first place, you enjoy good health. – Horace 65 BC

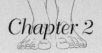

Chapter 2

Give Proper Loving Care To Your Feet That Carry You Through Life!

Clean Feet Are Important

Like the rest of your body, feet perspire. Each foot has thousands of sweat glands and because they're usually encased in shoes, socks or stockings, they retain more perspiration than less-restricted parts of the body. This can lead to unpleasant odors and accumulation of rough or dead skin that causes irritation and soreness.

You must tackle foot-bathing with real dedication and vigor. Keep the following items handy, right next to your tub or shower: a handbrush with moderately stiff bristles, a worn-out toothbrush and a pumice stone.

First, scrub your feet with the handbrush. Use health soaps (*tea tree, vegetable, herbal, oatmeal, glycerine, etc.*) and warm water. Do not neglect the soles of the feet. Next, scrub between the toes. Here is where you use the toothbrush, because these places are hard to get at otherwise. It's particularly important to get your feet absolutely clean because this helps to prevent athlete's foot, which is one of the most irritating of foot problems.

Now rinse feet and while they're still wet, if in shower sit down on shower stool and rub the pumice stone or foot file lightly on any foot parts that feel rough. This usually includes the heels and balls of feet. Use the stone with a gentle, rotary motion, as this helps to soften the skin and discourages heavy calluses from forming.

Drying your feet is very important. Athlete's foot is caused by a fungus that thrives on warm, damp skin. If you do not dry the foot thoroughly, especially between the toes, you are inviting this fungus which is difficult to overcome. Do not scrub-dry the areas between your toes. Pat them dry, gently but firmly. Otherwise, you may irritate these areas. The rest of the foot you may dry vigorously. In fact, this form of brief massage has the added advantage of stimulating foot circulation.

Pedicure and Trimming The Toenails

A good time to give yourself a pedicure is after your foot bath, when skin is warm and moist. You can gently push back the cuticle and rid toenails of excess cuticle that forms around nails. This habit prevents cuticles from growing wild. *(For salon pedicures be sure the instruments are sterilised or take your own.)*

When trimming your toenails, please never rip any off. This may leave a torn edge that can become extremely sensitive to shoe pressure. Also, never trim down into the corners of a nail as this is one of the chief causes of ingrown toenails. Trim the toenails straight across and leave the corners alone. Remember – ingrown toenails, corns, calluses, bunions and Athlete's Foot – all detract from the health, appearance and happiness of your feet!

Remember that the basic purpose of foot hygiene is to maintain a healthy tone and vigor in each foot, just as strengthening-up exercises are designed to keep the body trim. Hygienic foot-care is a routine habit that pays great dividends in healthier feet to carry you through life.

Finish off your pedicure with a massage using our Bragg Organic Extra Virgin Olive Oil to keep your feet flexible, soft and smooth. This oil is also great for the legs, arms, face and the entire body. (See web: www.bragg.com)

Baby Your Tired, Aching Feet

Tired, hurting feet can take the joy out of your life! This book is filled with ways to bring life back to your feet! Some methods are a little more elaborate than others, but all are just variations of foot care therapy: various special foot soaks (herbal, vinegar, Epsom salts), foot therapy, pedicure, massage, exercise and rest.

I cannot think clearly when my feet hurt!
– President Abraham Lincoln, 16th US President, 1861-1865

Remember the longest journey starts with just one step.

If you pick them up, O'Lord, I'll put'em down. – Prayer of Tired Walker

16

The average American has their feet encased in shoes for over 12 hours daily and most often the shoes are ill-fitting, resulting in foot problems.

Foot Bath and Foot Massage

The following special foot bath will prove beneficial. Sit on a chair next to the bathtub with your feet dangling under the tap. Turn on tap to make a strong flow for 5 to 10 minutes, alternating hot and cold water over feet (diabetic & heart patients caution using hot water: see pages 73, 75, 99). If you have a spray attachment, just spray alternating directly hot, then cold water, on your feet - feels so great!

After your foot bath, dry your feet thoroughly with a rough towel and be sure that all moisture is off the feet. Now sprinkle cornstarch over your feet and start your foot massage, using fingers, mainly thumbs, in a circular motion. Start on the bottoms of the feet. Put plenty of powder on your hands and massage the soles of your feet in rotary motion. With both hands, twist each foot back and forth in opposite directions to keep them limber and healthy. Then massage the sides and ankles in a rotary motion. Also, gently pull and twist each toe from its base. End up with a stroking massage motion. Don't be afraid to use pressure as this promotes more healthy blood circulation to the general structure of the feet and ankles, and helps wash the toxins and crystals out of the feet!

Please keep in mind that massage is very important in making the feet healthy, alive and tingling with vitality. Circulation reaches its weakest point in the feet because the heart has to drive blood down there; they are farthest from the heart and blood must flow against gravity to return to the heart. Hence, circulation may often become sluggish in the feet (cold and aching feet are two of the signs of poor circulation). See Chapter 11 (page 117) for more info on foot reflexology, a specialized and very pleasant, relaxing, powerful healing technique.

Every man is the builder of a temple called his body. We are all our own sculptors and painters and our material is our own flesh, blood and bones.
– Henry David Thoreau. Visit Web: www.eserver.org/thoreau
Dad and I loved our many visits to Walden Pond. Dad even duplicated Thoreau's Walden Pond Cabin for our retreat near Malibu, CA.

To our minds the greatest mistake a person can make is to remain ignorant when he is surrounded everyday of his life, with the knowledge he needs to grow and be healthy, happy and successful. It's all there – you need only observe, read, learn and then apply the wisdom.– Paul C. Bragg

17

Expert Advice on Banishing Athlete's Foot

Our body is normally the host to a variety of micro-organisms, including bacteria, mold-like fungi and yeast-like fungi. Some of these micro-organisms are useful to our body, but others may cause infections. Fungal skin infections are caused by microscopic fungi that can live on the skin. Athlete's Foot is the most common and most persistent of the fungal (tinea) infections. Athlete's Foot may occur in association with other fungal skin infections such as ringworm or jock itch. Mold-like fungi live on the dead tissues of the hair, nails and the outer skin layers and thrive in the warm, moist areas of the body.

Athlete's Foot is a skin disease caused by fungi which occurs usually between the toes. The fungus attacks the feet because shoes create a warm, moist environment which encourages its growth. Poor hygiene, prolonged moist skin and minor skin or nail injuries are also factors that can induce Athlete's Foot. Some symptoms to watch out for are: itching, stinging or burning, skin redness, rash or blisters, inflammation and discoloration and crumbling nails.

Athlete's Foot is contagious! It can be spread through items such as shoes, socks and shower and poolside surfaces of spas, clubs, summer camps, etc. Athlete's Foot may spread to the soles of the feet and toes, plus other body parts, notably the groin area and the underarms.

If you have Athlete's Foot, using self-care can help you banish the problem: Put 1/3 cup of Bragg Apple Cider Vinegar in shallow pan of warm water and soak feet once daily until gone (*ideal while reading or watching TV*); always keep feet clean and dry; always wear clean cotton or wool socks, change daily; wear shoes made of natural material such as leather, or canvas and best to alternate shoes daily. Shoes then have time to dry completely between wearings; reduce perspiration by using cornstarch powder. When you are infected with Athlete's Foot, it's good to change bed sheets and clothing often to prevent the infection from spreading. For more Athlete's Foot info see these additional pages 15,18,79,80,108,111,112,115,135.

All the flowers of all the tomorrows are in the seeds of today.

Love is living in harmony with yourself and all those around you and all that surrounds you. – Amrit Desai

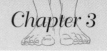

Chapter 3

Your Posture and Your Feet

Perfect Posture Promotes Perfect Feet

Why should emphasis be placed upon such a simple thing as the pull of gravity? This is very easy to explain. In youth, as long as your muscles were strong enough, they held your skeleton in proper balance with its many points and sections free from strain or discomfort. As your body ages, your muscles start to lose the battle with gravity, especially if you are prematurely ageing or heavier than you should be, or a forced rest has weakened your muscles just enough to cause an uncomfortable state of body imbalance. Slumping stretches your back's ligaments and causes backaches. Ligaments are meant to serve only as check reins for the joints and they cannot be forcibly stretched without, in time, causing pain.

When the ligaments in your back are made stiff and uncomfortable by this, it's only natural for your muscles to try to oppose this sagging of your back which results from the pull of gravity (poor posture). However, when your muscles are too weak to do their job, they rapidly become exhausted and develop fatigue, making good posture impossible and your back even more uncomfortable!

Check your own posture and symptoms (see page 23). Do you notice a deep aching and soreness along your spine due to stretched ligaments? Are your back and shoulder areas achy and tired? Is your backache due basically to weak muscles? If it is, it's about time you did something sensible to relieve it, like strengthening all those weak muscles by proper exercise and posture.

Do not pray for a lighter pack; simply ask for a stronger back.

Our habits, good or bad, are something we can control. – Dr. E. J. Stieglitz

---

Happiness is a rainbow in your heart – a health sparkler! – Patricia Bragg

The Mirror Never Lies

Look at yourself in the mirror! Do your shoulders slump? Is your upper back round? Is your chest bowed in? Have you a potbelly? Are you swaybacked? Can you see the reasons now why your back has a right to ache? The bending, slumping, ligament-stretching force of gravity has finally taken charge. But even if you are presently suffering backaches due to poor muscles and bad posture habits, don't despair. You can regain back comfort if weak muscles and poor posture are at fault!

It's been said that backache is the penalty man must pay for the privilege of standing and walking upright on two feet. Although man's ancestors are believed by some (not the authors) to have been four-footed creatures, there is no doubt about the fact that man himself is definitely two-footed! Every infant struggles instinctively to stand on his own two feet and walk! He needs not be taught! He will attempt his biped gait even if left alone most of the time and never instructed. It is natural for a human being to stand and walk in this manner! This is interesting, because there are no animals which spend all of their standing and walking hours on two feet, not even the chimpanzees or the gorillas. These higher apes use their hands and arms to help them about. The world's strongest gorilla would be unable to follow a fragile housewife about, walking as erectly as she does, for more than a short time. This is because human beings are meant to walk erect, and animals are not!

Strong Muscles Help Make Strong Spine

Human spines have normal curves which enable the muscles to oppose gravity and hold the back erect. As long as the muscles are strong enough to maintain the balance of these curves and prevent sagging, the back is comfortable. When the muscles are too weak to do this normal work, the back sags, ligaments are stretched, and then backache enters the picture. Remember to maintain one's body in a healthy state involves many factors: healthy foods, rest, exercise, sleep, fasting, control of emotions and mind and, last but not least, good posture.

If a body is well-nourished and cared for, good posture is not a problem. When the body lacks the essentials, poor posture is often the result. Once poor lifestyle habits have been established, one must change to definite, corrective healthy lifestyle living, such as proper exercises and daily deliberate healthy postural habits, etc.

How to Stand Erect and Walk for Health

When walking, one should imagine that the legs are attached to the middle of the chest. This gives long, sweeping, graceful, springy steps, because when one walks correctly with this full swing and spring, one automatically builds energy. Habits either make or break us, and good posture habits make graceful, strong bodies.

. . . Just as the twig is bent, the tree is inclined.

POSTURE SILHOUETTES: Which one are you?

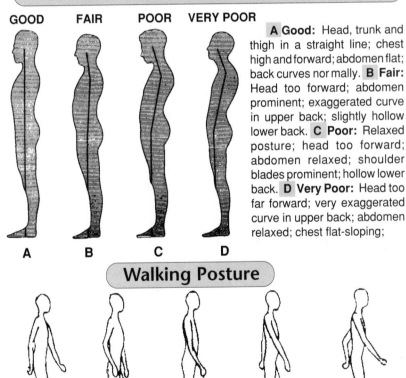

GOOD   FAIR   POOR   VERY POOR

A Good: Head, trunk and thigh in a straight line; chest high and forward; abdomen flat; back curves normally. **B Fair:** Head too forward; abdomen prominent; exaggerated curve in upper back; slightly hollow lower back. **C Poor:** Relaxed posture; head too forward; abdomen relaxed; shoulder blades prominent; hollow lower back. **D Very Poor:** Head too far forward; very exaggerated curve in upper back; abdomen relaxed; chest flat-sloping;

A   B   C   D

Walking Posture

Always prepare a new base before leaving the old.

Bragg Posture Exercises
Promote Health and Youthfulness

Looking in the mirror, stand tall, feet 8" apart, tighten butt and suck in stomach muscles, lift up rib cage, stretch up spine, chest out, shoulders back, chin up slightly, line body up straight (nose plumbline straight to belly button), drop hands (heavy) to sides and swing your arms back and forth to normalize your posture. Do this posture exercise daily and miraculous changes will happen! You are now retraining and strengthening your muscles to stand straight for health and youthfulness! Remember when you slump, you also cramp your precious machinery. This posture exercise will retrain your frame to sit, stand and walk tall for supreme health, fitness and increase your longevity!

When in sitting position, see that the spine is stretched up and have your back against chair so that the abdominal cavity is not relaxed, but drawn in some. Have your shoulders back, with head held high, never jutting forward. Have arms and hands relaxed in lap. Never clasp arms (vice-like) around your chest, this bad habit impedes your circulation.

Don't Sit With Your Legs Crossed – It's A Killer!

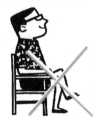

Remember when in a sitting position, never cross one leg over the other. Under the knees run two of the largest arteries, carrying nourishing blood to the muscles below the knee and to the thousands of nerves in the legs and feet. When you cross your legs, you immediately cut down the blood flow to almost a trickle. Then, when the leg and the knee muscles are not nourished and don't have good circulation, the body starts going stagnant in the extremities, this can lead to broken capillaries, varicose veins and other health problems. Look at the bare ankles and legs of people over 40 who made a habit of crossing their legs and see their problems. Also when the muscles and feet don't get their full blood supply, the feet become weak and poor circulation and stagnation sets in. Cold feet torment most leg-crossers.

A well-known heart specialist was asked once, *"When do most people have a heart attack?"* The heart specialist answered, *"At a time when they are sitting quietly with one leg crossed over the other."* So now you can see that when you sit down you should put both feet squarely on the floor and remember never again cross your legs!!!

WHERE DO YOU STAND?

POSTURE CHART

	PERFECT	FAIR	POOR
HEAD			
SHOULDERS			
SPINE			
HIPS			
ANKLES			
NECK			
UPPER BACK			
TRUNK			
ABDOMEN			
LOWER BACK			

Your posture carries you through life from your head to your feet. This is your human vehicle and you are truly a miracle! Cherish, respect and always protect it by living The Bragg Healthy Lifestyle. – Patricia Bragg

23

Remember – Your posture can make or break your health!

Poor Posture Promotes Pain and Ageing

People who are habitual leg-crossers always have more acid crystals stored in the feet than those who never cross their legs while sitting. Crossing the legs is one of the worst postural habits of man, it stresses and burdens the heart! It throws the hips, spine and head off balance and is one of the main causes of chronic backache!

Poor posture of any kind can bring you unbearable pain across your upper back and fatigue in your drooping shoulders, as well as soreness shooting from the base of your neck to the back and downward to mingle with stiffness in the waist and hip area of your lower back. Poor posture can cause weakness in the hips and loins, a numb feeling at your tailbone, and a shooting pain down your legs. Bad posture can develop aches and pains not only in the back and feet, but all over the body!

One very simple habit, but a most beneficial one to establish, is to stand tall, walk tall, sit tall, and never cross one leg over the other! This does not require an exaggerated position. When one stands tall, walks tall and sits tall, a correct posture is assumed and all of the sagging, and prolapsed vital organs will soon assume normal position and better functioning — that is, if all other healthy habits of living are practiced daily as well.

The Correct Way to Sit in Chairs

Standing, walking, sitting and getting up from the sitting position must be done correctly in order to promote the correct use of the feet, the knee joints and the hip joints. We want you to pay particular attention to these instructions on how to sit and how to get up from a chair. The greater majority of humans, when they sit in a chair, they flop themselves into it. Or, instead of using the movable body joints, they use the chair arms to get into and out of it. In doing this they are not using the feet, knee or hip joints properly. Years of flopping into a chair and using the arms of the chair to get out have caused the bones of the feet, the knees and the hip joints to deteriorate. Not only is damage done to these members of the body, but the flopping into the chair shocks all 24 movable bones of the spine. This can slowly wear away the discs between the vertebrae and bones of the spine. Soon bones are pressing upon bones, impinging on and damaging nerves that affect many parts of the body adversely.

Make Your Mind Your Health Captain

First you must use your mind to direct your body. We are believers in healthy constructive, conscious control of the body. All moves should be first thought out before they are executed. Most people move their bodies without any conscious direction and this is the reason their bodies, particularly their posture, feet and spine deteriorate and bring on grave and painful physical problems.

Before you sit in a chair, think of how you are going to sit in that chair properly. To learn this technique, think of yourself as a puppet with a string attached to the center of your skull. Now you are going to lower yourself carefully, lightly and gently into that chair just as though you were a puppet being moved up and down gently. First start with your head, which should be forward and up, your neck should be relaxed, the spine is to be made long and the lower part of your back is widened. We are going to use the hip joints as the big hinges for sitting down. As you lower the hips you should bend forward like a jackknife being closed and, using the power that is in the feet, the ankles, the knees and hips gently and lightly lower yourself into the seat. The back should sit well back in the chair, and be supported by the chair back. So, before you sit down, keep these pertinent facts in mind: head forward and up, back lengthening and bend forward as you sit down as though the blade of a jackknife is being closed, then opened when you sit.

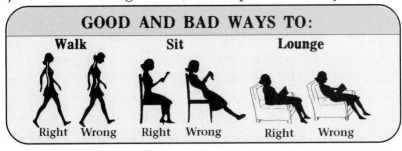

GOOD AND BAD WAYS TO:

Walk — Right Wrong Sit — Right Wrong Lounge — Right Wrong

25

Now to get yourself out of the chair. Contemplate how you are going to get out of the chair and do it correctly. Give yourself the instructions again: head forward and up, back lengthening and widening, close the jackknife as you rise from the chair, and when you are in the full standing position the jackknife is open. If you will continue to do this every time you sit down and get up, you will find that your feet are going to be stronger. They are going to have more strength because you are using them correctly. Remember, we told you there are 26 movable bones in each foot and you must protect them and use them wisely!

What You Don't Exercise and Use – You Lose!

Paul C. Bragg repeatedly stated, to maintain good health the body must be exercised properly (walking, jogging, biking, swimming, deep breathing, stretching, calisthenics, good posture, etc.) and nourished wisely (healthy natural foods), so as to provide and increase the good life of radiant health, joy and happiness.

Lifting Posture

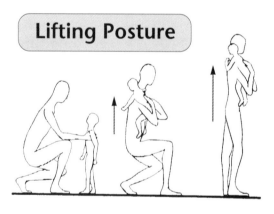

Lifting weight: The weight of the baby is held close to the center of gravity directly above the pushing force.

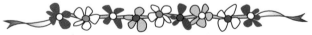

25% of the body's bones are in the feet.

Women have four times as many foot problems as men do.

You cannot put the same shoe on every foot. – Pubilius Syrus

The civilized man has built cars, but has lost the use of his feet. – Emerson

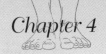

Chapter 4

The Importance of Healthy Nutrition

Strong, sturdy, enduring, tireless, painless, ageless feeling feet are built by a healthy well-nourished, rich, red bloodstream. Your blood is made from the food you eat and the liquids you drink.

Every 90 days you build a complete new bloodstream. So in 90 days, with careful attention to your food program, you can build a bloodstream that is going to help you cleanse, heal and rebuild new, strong, healthy feet.

To build strong feet and a healthy bloodstream, let's first discuss what *not* to do. The worst enemies of healthy feet and blood are white refined sugars, white refined flours, white rice, alcohol, tobacco, coffee, tea and all the soft drinks! It is impossible to build a healthy, rich bloodstream, and maintain healthy feet and body out of these unhealthy, toxic materials. No building is built with poor materials; large cities have strict building ordinances that require building materials of the highest quality. Your health is your greatest wealth! Don't let your body prematurely age and decay! Apply strict specifications and the best quality body building materials possible. Your body is a miracle instrument and please regard it as such! You should only put into your body foods that build healthy, strong bones and tendons in all the movable joints of the feet, legs and body.

A good nutritious diet is based on the amount of protective foods that are used in it. For a healthy diet have ample raw and properly cooked organic vegetables and fresh fruits (page 29). Also have a balance of protein *(vegetarian is best)*, plus minerals, vitamins and enzymes.

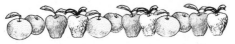

You are what you eat, drink, breathe, think, say and do!
– Patricia Bragg, N.D., Ph.D., Health Crusader

BENEFITS FROM THE JOYS OF FASTING

Fasting renews your faith in yourself, your strength and Gods strength.
Fasting is easier than any diet. • Fasting is the quickest way to lose weight.
Fasting is adaptable to a busy life. • Fasting gives the body a physiological rest.
Fasting is used successfully in the treatment of many physical illnesses.
Fasting can yield weight losses of up to 10 pounds or more in the first week.
Fasting lowers & normalizes cholesterol, homocysteine & blood pressure levels.
Fasting improves dietary habits. • Fasting increases pleasure eating healthy foods.
Fasting is a calming experience, often relieving tension and insomnia.
Fasting frequently induces feelings of euphoria, a natural high.
Fasting is a miracle rejuvenator, slowing the ageing process.
Fasting is a natural stimulant to rejuvenate the growth hormone levels.
Fasting is an energizer, not a debilitator. • Fasting aids the elimination process.
Fasting often results in a more vigorous marital relationship.
Fasting can eliminate smoking, drug and drinking addictions.
Fasting is a regulator, educating the body to consume food only as needed.
Fasting saves time spent marketing, preparing and eating.
Fasting rids the body of toxins, giving it an internal shower & cleansing.
Fasting does not deprive the body of essential nutrients.
Fasting can be used to uncover the sources of food allergies.
Fasting is used effectively in schizrenia treatment & other mental illnesses.
Fasting under proper supervision can be tolerated easily up to four weeks.
Fasting does not accumulate appetite; hunger pangs disappear in 1-2 days.
Fasting is routine for the animal kingdom.
Fasting has been a common practice since the beginning of man's existence.
Fasting is a rite in all religions; the Bible alone has 74 references to it.
Fasting under proper conditions is absolutely safe. • Fasting is a blessing.
Fasting is not starving, it's nature's cure that God has given us. – Patricia Bragg
                    – Allan Cott, M.D., *Fasting As A Way Of Life*

Spiritual Bible Reasons Why We Should Fast

Acts 13:2-3	Deut. 11:7-14,21	Luke 4:2-5,14	Matthew 9: 9-15
Acts 14:23-25	Ezra 8:23	Luke 9:1-6,11	Matthew 17:18-21
3 John 2	Gen. 6:3	Mark 2:16-20	Neh. 1:4
1 Cor. 10:31	Gal. 5:16-26	Matthew 4:1-4	Neh. 9:1, 20-21
1 Cor. 13:4-7	Isaiah 58:6,8	Matthew 6:16-18	Psalms 35:13
Deut. 8:3-8	Joel 2:12	Matthew 7:7-8	Psalms 119:18

Dear Health Friend,

This gentle reminder explains the great benefits from *The Miracle of Fasting* that you will enjoy when starting on your weekly 24 hour Bragg Fasting Program for Super Health! It's a precious time of body-mind-soul cleansing and renewal.

On fast days I drink 8 to 10 glasses of distilled (our favorite) or purified water, (I add 1-2 tsps Bragg Organic Vinegar to 3 of them). If just starting, you may also try herbal teas or try diluted fresh juices with $1/3$ distilled water. Every day, even some fast days, add 1 Tbsp of psyllium husk powder to liquids once daily. It's an extra cleanser and helps normalize weight, cholesterol and blood pressure and helps promote healthy elimination. Fasting is the oldest, most effective healing method known to man. Fasting offers great, miraculous blessings from Mother Nature and our Creator. It begins the self-cleansing of the inner-body workings so we can promote our own self-healing.

My father and I wrote the book *The Miracle of Fasting* to share with you the health miracles it can perform in your life. It's all so worthwhile to do and it's an important part of The Bragg Healthy Lifestyle.

With Love, *Patricia*

Paul Bragg's work on fasting and water is one of the great contributions to The Healing Wisdom and The Natural Health Movement in the world today.
– Gabriel Cousens, M.D., Author of Conscious Eating & Spiritual Nutrition

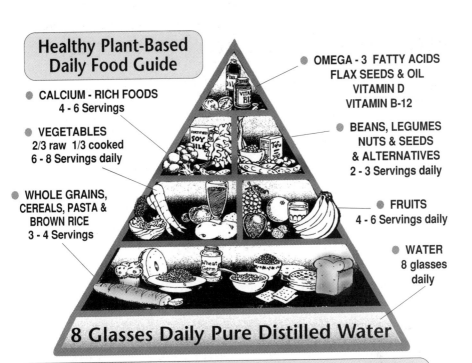

Healthy Plant-Based Daily Food Guide

- **CALCIUM - RICH FOODS**
  4 - 6 Servings

- **VEGETABLES**
  2/3 raw 1/3 cooked
  6 - 8 Servings daily

- **WHOLE GRAINS, CEREALS, PASTA & BROWN RICE**
  3 - 4 Servings

- **OMEGA - 3 FATTY ACIDS FLAX SEEDS & OIL VITAMIN D VITAMIN B-12**

- **BEANS, LEGUMES NUTS & SEEDS & ALTERNATIVES**
  2 - 3 Servings daily

- **FRUITS**
  4 - 6 Servings daily

- **WATER**
  8 glasses daily

8 Glasses Daily Pure Distilled Water

Warning! – Avoid All Unhealthy Microwaved Foods!

In the past 25 years microwaves have practically replaced traditional methods of cooking, especially with on-the-go people of today's world. But how much do you really know about them? Are they no more than timesaving machines for cooking? A Swiss Study found that food which is microwaved is not the food it was before! The microwave radiation deforms and destroys the molecular structure of the food – creating radiolytic compounds! When microwaved food is eaten, abnormal changes occur in your blood and immune systems. These include a decrease in hemoglobin and white blood cell counts and an increase in cholesterol levels. An article in Pediatrics Journal warns microwaving human milk damages the anti-infective properties it usually gives to a mother's baby. Research work done by The University of Warwick in Great Britain warns that microwave radiation is very damaging to the vital electromagnetic activity of human life vibrations. See web: warwick.ac.uk/news/pr/97. Over 20 years ago Russia established wise microwave radiation limits more stringent than United States and Great Britain. Beware, don't use microwaves!! See web: relfe.com/microwave.html

Aspartame – Artificial Diet Sweetener Unhealthy & Makes You Fat!

*Because Monsanto's artificial sweetener Aspartame (sold as "Nutrasweet," "Equal," and "Spoonful") is over 200 times sweeter than sugar, it's a common ingredient in "diet" foods and has become a sweetening staple for dieters. Besides being a deadly poison, aspartame actually contributes to weight gain by causing a craving for carbohydrates. Study of 80,000 women by American Cancer Society found those who used this neurotoxic "diet" sweetener actually gained more weight than those who didn't use aspartame products. Read more health risks on web: aspartamekills.com. **Herb Stevia sweetener is a healthy alternative**.*

Food and Product Summary

Today, many of our foods are highly processed or refined, robbing them of essential nutrients, vitamins, minerals and enzymes. Many also contain harmful, toxic and dangerous chemicals. The research findings and experience of top nutritionists, physicians and dentists have led to the discovery that devitalized foods are major causes of poor health, illness, cancer and premature death. The enormous increase in the last 70 years of degenerative diseases such as heart disease, arthritis and dental decay substantiate this belief. Scientific research has shown that most of these can be prevented and others, can be arrested or even reversed through improved nutrition and lifestyle changes.

Enjoy Super Health with Natural Foods

1. **RAW FOODS:** Fresh fruits and raw vegetables organically grown are always best. Enjoy nutritious variety garden salads with raw vegetables, sprouts, raw nuts and seeds.

2. **VEGETABLES and PROTEINS:**
   a. Legumes, lentils, brown rice, soy beans, and all beans.
   b. Nuts and seeds, raw and unsalted.
   c. We prefer healthier vegetarian proteins. If you must have animal protein, then be sure it's hormone–free, and organically fed and no more than 1 or 2 times a week.
   d. Dairy products – fresh fertile range-free eggs are best, unprocessed hard cheese and feta goat's cheese. We choose not to use dairy products. Try the healthier non-dairy soy, rice, nut, and almond milks and soy cheeses, yogurt and occasionally soy or rice ice cream.

3. **FRUITS and VEGETABLES:** Organically grown is always best – grown without the use of poisonous sprays and toxic chemical fertilizers whenever possible; urge your market to stock organic produce! Steam, bake, sauté or wok vegetables as short a time as possible to retain the best nutritional content and flavor. Also enjoy fresh juices.

4. **100% WHOLE GRAIN CEREALS, BREADS and FLOURS:** They contain important B-complex vitamins, vitamin E, minerals, fiber and the important unsaturated fatty acids.

5. **COLD, EXPELLER – PRESSED HEALTHY OILS:** Bragg organic extra virgin olive & macadamia oils are best, rich in oleic acid. Also soy, flax & sesame oils are excellent sources of healthy essential oils. We still use oils sparingly.

USA leads the world in heart disease, strokes, cancer and diabetes! Why? It's our fast junk foods, high sugars, fats, milk and processed foods diet.

If just half of the $billions spent on cancer research were spent on educating the public how to avoid disease - millions of lives would be saved from cancer.
– Joel Fuhrman, M.D., Author, Fasting and Eating for Health

HEALTHY BEVERAGES
Fresh Juices, Herb Teas & Pep Drinks

These freshly squeezed organic vegetable and fruit juices are important to The Bragg Healthy Lifestyle. It's not wise to drink beverages with your main meals, as it dilutes the digestive juices. But it's great during the day to have a glass of freshly squeezed orange, grapefruit, vegetable juice, Bragg Vinegar ACV Drink, herb tea or try hot cup Bragg Liquid Aminos Broth (½ to 1 tsp Bragg Liquid Aminos in cup of hot distilled water) – these are all ideal pick-me-up beverages.

Bragg Apple Cider Vinegar Cocktail – Mix 1-2 tsps equally of Bragg Organic ACV and (optional) raw honey, blackstrap molasses or pure maple syrup in 8 oz. distilled or purified water. Take glass upon arising, hour before lunch and dinner (*if diabetic, to sweeten use 2-4 stevia drops*).

Delicious Hot or Cold Cider Drink – Add 2 to 3 cinnamon sticks and 4 cloves to water and boil. Steep 20 minutes or more. Before serving add Bragg Vinegar and raw honey to taste. (*Re-use cinnamon sticks & cloves*)

Bragg Favorite Juice Cocktail – This drink consists of all raw vegetables (please remember organic is best) which we prepare in our vegetable juicer: carrots, celery, beets, cabbage, tomatoes, watercress and parsley, etc. The great purifier, garlic, we enjoy but it's optional.

Bragg Favorite Health Smoothie "Pep" Drink – After morning stretch and exercises we often enjoy this drink instead of fruit. It's delicious and powerfully nutritious as a meal anytime: lunch, dinner or take in thermos to work, school, sports, gym, hiking, and to park or freeze for popsicles.

Bragg Health Smoothie "Pep" Drink

Prepare following in blender, add frozen juice cube if desired colder; Choice of: freshly squeezed orange or grapefruit juice; carrot and greens juice; unsweetened pineapple juice; or 1½ - 2 cups purified or distilled water with:

2 tsps spirulina or green powder, barley, etc.	1 to 2 bananas, ripe
2 tsp raw wheat germ (optional)	1 tsp soy protein powder
2 Tbsp flax oil (or grind Tbsp of flax seeds)	1 tsp sunflower or chia seeds
2 tsp lecithin granules	1 tsp raw honey (optional)
1 tsp rice or oat bran	1 tsp vit C or emer'gen-C powder
2 tsp psyllium husk powder (optional)	2 tsp nutritional yeast flakes
2 dates or prunes, pitted (optional)	3 cup soy yogurt or tofu

Optional: 8 apricots (sundried, unsulphured) soak in jar overnight in purified water or unsweetened pineapple juice. We soak enough for several days, keep refrigerated – also delicious topped with soy yogurt . Add seasonal organic fresh fruit: peaches, strawberries, berries, apricots, etc. instead of banana. In winter, add apples, kiwi, oranges, tangelos, persimmons or pears, and if fresh is unavailable, try sugar-free, frozen organic fruits. Servings 1 to 2.

Patricia's Delicious Health Popcorn

Use freshly popped organic popcorn (use air popper). Try Bragg Organic Olive, Macadamia, Flax Oil or melted salt-free butter over popcorn. Add several sprays Bragg Aminos and Bragg Apple Cider Vinegar. . . Yes – it's delicious! Now sprinkle with nutritional yeast (large) flakes. For variety try pinch of Italian or French herbs, cayenne pepper, mustard powder or fresh crushed garlic to oil mixture. Serve instead of breads!

Bragg Lentil & Brown Rice Casserole, Burgers or Soup
Jack LaLanne's Favorite Recipe

14 oz pkg lentils, uncooked　　　*12　cups brown organic rice, uncooked*
4 - 6 carrots, chop 1" rounds　　　　*or substitute grains of choice*
2 onions, chop, (optional)　　　　*1 tsp Bragg Liquid Aminos*
4 garlic cloves, chop, (optional)　*4　tsp Italian herbs (oregano, basil, etc.)*
2-3 quarts, distilled water　　　　*2 tsps Bragg Organic Extra Virgin Olive Oil*

Wash & drain lentils & rice. Place grains in large stainless steel pot. Add water, bring to boil, reduce heat, then add vegetables & seasonings to grains and simmer for 30 minutes. If desired, last 5 minutes add fresh or canned (salt-free) tomatoes before serving. For delicious garnish add spray of Bragg Aminos, minced parsley & nutritional yeast (large) flakes. Mash or blend for burgers. For soup, add more water. Serves 4 to 6.

Bragg Raw Organic Vegetable Health Salad

2 stalks celery, chop　　　　　*½ cup red cabbage, chop*
1 bell pepper & seeds, dice　　*½ cup alfalfa or sunflower sprouts*
½ cucumber, slice　　　　　　*2 spring onions & green tops, chop*
2 carrots, grate　　　　　　　*1 turnip, grate*
1 raw beet, grate　　　　　　*1 avocado (ripe)*
1 cup green cabbage, slice　　*3 tomatoes, medium size*

For variety add organic raw zucchini, sugar peas, mushrooms, broccoli, cauliflower (try black olives & pasta). Chop, slice or grate vegetables fine to medium for variety in size. Mix vegetables & serve on bed of lettuce, spinach, watercress or chopped cabbage. Dice avocado & tomato & serve on side as a dressing. Serve choice of fresh squeezed lemon, orange or dressing separately. Chill salad plates before serving. **It's best to always eat salad first before serving hot dishes.** Serves 3 to 5.

Bragg Health Salad Dressing

½ cup Bragg Organic Apple Cider Vinegar　　*½ tsp Bragg Liquid Aminos*
1-2 tsps organic raw honey to taste　　　　*1-2 cloves garlic, mince*
⅓ cup Bragg Organic Olive Oil, or blend with macadamia, soy, sesame or flax oil
1 Tbsp fresh herbs, minced or pinch of Italian or French dry herbs

Blend ingredients in blender or jar. Refrigerate in covered jar.

FOR DELICIOUS HERBAL VINEGAR: In quart jar add ⅓ cup tightly packed, crushed fresh sweet basil, tarragon, dill, oregano, or any fresh herbs desired, combined or singly. (If *dried* herbs, use 1-2 tsps herbs.) Now cover to top with Bragg Organic Apple Cider Vinegar and store two weeks in warm place, and then strain and refrigerate.

Honey – Celery Seed Vinaigrette

½ tsp dry mustard　　　　　*1 cup Bragg Organic Apple Cider Vinegar*
1 tsp Bragg Liquid Aminos　*½ cup Bragg Organic Extra Virgin Olive Oil*
¼ tsp paprika　　　　　　　*1 tsp celery seed*
⅓ cup raw honey to taste　　*1 tsp fresh ginger, peeled, mash*

Blend ingredients in blender or jar. Refrigerate in covered jar.

Avoid These Processed, Refined, Harmful Foods

Once you realize the harm caused to your body by unhealthy, refined, chemicalized, deficient foods, you'll want to eliminate these "killer" foods. Also avoid microwaved foods! Follow The Bragg Healthy Lifestyle to provide the basic, healthy nourishment to maintain your health.

- Refined sugar, artificial sweeteners (toxic aspartame) or their products such as jams, jellies, preserves, marmalades, yogurts, ice cream, sherbets, Jello, cake, candy, cookies, all chewing gum, colas & diet drinks, pies, pastries, and all sugared fruit juices & fruits canned in sugar syrup. **(Health Stores have healthy delicious replacements, Stevia, etc, so seek and buy the best.)**

- White flour products such as white bread, wheat-white bread, enriched flours, rye bread that has white flour in it, dumplings, biscuits, buns, gravy, pasta, pancakes, waffles, soda crackers, pizza, ravioli, pies, pastries, cakes, cookies, prepared and commercial puddings and ready-mix bakery products. Most made with dangerous (oxy-cholesterol) powdered milk and powdered eggs. **(Health Stores have huge variety of 100% whole grain organic products, delicious breads, crackers, pastas, desserts, etc.)**

- Salted foods, such as corn chips, potato chips, pretzels, crackers and nuts.

- Refined white rices and pearled barley. • Fast fried foods. • Indian ghee.

- Refined, sugared (also, aspartame), dry processed cereals – cornflakes, etc.

- Foods that contain olestra, palm and cottonseed oil. These additives are not fit for human consumption and should be totally avoided.

- Peanuts and peanut butter that contain hydrogenated, hardened oils and any peanut mold and all molds that can cause allergies.

- Margarine – combines heart-deadly trans-fatty acids and saturated fats.

- Saturated fats and hydrogenated oils – enemies that clog the arteries.

- Coffee, decaffeinated coffee, caffeinated tea and all alcoholic beverages. Also all caffeinated and sugared water-juices, all cola and soft drinks.

- Fresh pork and products.• Fried, fatty meats.• Irradiated and GMO foods.

- Smoked meats, such as ham, bacon, sausage and smoked fish.

- Luncheon meats, hot dogs, salami, bologna, corned beef, pastrami and packaged meats containing dangerous sodium nitrate or nitrite.

- Dried fruits containing sulphur dioxide – a toxic preservative.

- Don't eat chickens or turkeys that have been injected with hormones or fed with commercial poultry feed containing any drugs or toxins.

- Canned soups - read labels for sugar, salt, starch, flour and preservatives.

- Foods containing benzoate of soda, salt, sugar, cream of tartar and any additives, drugs, preservatives; irradiated and genetically engineered foods.

- Day-old cooked vegetables, potatoes and pre-mixed, wilted lifeless salads.

- All commercial vinegars: pasteurized, filtered, distilled, white, malt and synthetic vinegars are dead vinegars! *(We use only our Bragg Organic Raw, Unfiltered Apple Cider Vinegar with the "Mother Enzyme" as used in olden times.)*

Enjoy Healthy Fiber for Super Health

- KEEP BEANS HANDY, probably the best fiber sources. Cook dried beans and freeze in portions. Use canned beans for faster meals.
- EAT BERRIES, surprisingly good sources of fiber.
- INSTEAD OF ICEBERG LETTUCE, choose deep green lettuces, romaine, bib, butter, etc., spinach or cabbage for variety salads.
- LOOK FOR "100% WHOLE WHEAT" and organic whole grain breads. A dark color isn't proof; check labels, compare fibers, grains, etc.
- WHOLE GRAIN CEREALS. Hot and cold granolas with sliced fruit.
- GO FOR BROWN RICE. It's better for you and so delicious.
- EAT THE SKINS of potatoes and other organic fruits and vegetables.
- LOOK FOR HEALTH CRACKERS with at least 2 grams of fiber per ounce.
- SERVE HUMMUS, made from chickpeas, instead of sour-cream dips.
- USE WHOLE WHEAT FLOUR for baking breads, muffins, pastries, pancakes, waffles and for variety try other whole grain flours.
- ADD OAT BRAN, WHEAT BRAN AND WHEATGERM to baked goods, cookies, etc.; whole grain cereals, casseroles, loafs, etc.
- SNACK ON SUN-DRIED FRUIT, such as apricots, dates, prunes, raisins, etc., which are concentrated sources of nutrients and fiber.
- INSTEAD OF DRINKING JUICE, eat fresh fruit: orange, grapefruit, apples, bananas, etc.; and vegetables: tomato, carrot, cabbage, etc.
  – UC Berkeley WellnessLetter (*www.berkeleywellness.com*)

Bad Nutrition – #1 Cause of Sickness

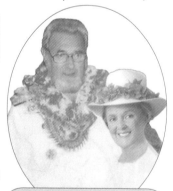

Dr. Koop & Patricia

People don't die of infectious conditions as such, but of malnutrition that allows the germs to gain a foothold in sickly bodies. Bad nutrition is usually one of the main causes of noninfectious, degenerative or fatal conditions. When the body has its full vitamin and mineral quota, including precious potassium, it is impossible for germs to get a foothold in its healthy bloodstream and tissues! We greatly admire our friend, the former U.S. Surgeon General Dr. C. Everett Koop who, in his famous 1988 landmark report on nutrition and health, stated this strong statement:

Diet-related diseases account for 68% of all United States deaths!

Vegetarian Protein % Chart

LEGUMES	%
Soybean Sprouts	54
Soybean Curd (tofu)	43
Soy flour	35
Soybeans	35
Broad Beans	32
Lentils	29
Split Peas	28
Kidney Beans	26
Navy Beans	26
Lima Beans	26
Garbanzo Beans	23

VEGETABLES	%
Spirulina *(Plant Algae)*	60
Spinach	49
New Zealand Spinach	47
Watercress	46
Kale	45
Broccoli	45
Brussels Sprouts	44
Turnip Greens	43
Collards	43
Cauliflower	40
Mustard Greens	39
Mushrooms	38
Chinese Cabbage	34
Parsley	34
Lettuce	34
Green Peas	30
Zucchini	28
Green Beans	26
Cucumbers	24
Dandelion Greens	24
Green Pepper	22
Artichokes	22
Cabbage	22
Celery	21
Eggplant	21
Tomatoes	18
Onions	16
Beets	15
Pumpkin	12
Potatoes	11
Yams	8
Sweet Potatoes	6

GRAINS	%
Wheat Germ	31
Rye	20
Wheat, hard red	17
Wild rice	16
Buckwheat	15
Oatmeal	15
Millet	12
Barley	11
Brown Rice	8

FRUITS	%
Lemons	16
Honeydew Melon	10
Cantaloupe	9
Strawberry	8
Orange	8
Blackberry	8
Cherry	8
Apricot	8
Grape	8
Watermelon	8
Tangerine	7
Papaya	6
Peach	6
Pear	5
Banana	5
Grapefruit	5
Pineapple	3
Apple	1

NUTS AND SEEDS	%
Pumpkin Seeds	21
Sunflower Seeds	17
Walnuts, black	13
Sesame Seeds	13
Almonds	12
Cashews	12
Macadamias	9

Data obtained from Nutritive Value of American Foods in Common Units, USDA Agriculture Handbook No. 456. Reprinted with author's permission, from *Diet for a New America* by John Robbins Available online on Amazon.com

Vitamin E Antioxidant Heart Healthy Foods Are Important for Your Health & Longevity

A partial list of foods that contain the following amounts of precious, healthy Vitamin E. This list was compiled from *The Bridges Food and Beverage Analysis.*

Food	Quantity	Vitamin E IU's
Apples	1 medium	0.74
Bananas	1 medium	0.40
Barley	½ cup	4.20
Beans, Navy	½ cup	3.60
Butter (salt-free)	2 tablespoons	0.80
Carrots	1 cup	0.45
Celery, Green	½ cup	2.60
Corn, Dried for Popcorn	1 cup	20.00
Cornmeal, Yellow	1 cup	3.40
Corn Oil	2 tablespoons	29.00
Eggs, Fertile	2	2.00
Endive, Escarole	½ cup	2.00
Flour, Whole Grain	1 cup	54.00
Grapefruit	½	0.52
Kale	½ cup	8.00
Lettuce	6 leaves	0.50
Oatmeal	½ cup	2.00
Olive Oil (virgin)	½ cup	5.00
Onions, Raw	2 medium	0.26
Oranges	1 small	0.24
Parsley	½ cup	5.50
Peas, Green	1 cup	4.00
Potatoes, White	1 medium	0.06
Potatoes, Sweet	1 small	4.00
Rice, Brown	1 cup cooked	2.40
Rye	½ cup	3.00
Soybean Oil	2 tablespoons	46.00
Sunflower Seeds, Raw	½ cup	31.00
Wheatgerm Oil	2 tablespoons	140.00

Plus E's in seeds, raw nuts, spinach, broccoli, avocados, etc. also in cooked beans.

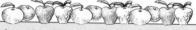

Bragg Vegetarian Recipe Book Has 100's of Delicious Healthy Salads, Soups, Casseroles, Desserts, etc.

Latest National Cancer Institute Research and Studies show Vitamin E and improving nutrition with fresh vegetables & fruit reduces cancer risk rates.

THE MIRACLES OF APPLE CIDER VINEGAR FOR A STRONGER, LONGER, HEALTHIER LIFE

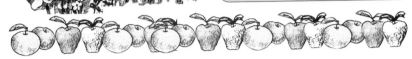

> The old adage is true:
> *"An apple a day
> keeps the doctor away."*

- Helps promote a youthful skin and vibrant healthy body
- Helps remove artery plaque and body toxins
- Helps fight germs, viruses, bacteria and mold naturally
- Helps retard old age onset in humans, pets and farm animals
- Helps regulate calcium metabolism
- Helps keep blood the right consistency
- Helps regulate women's menstruation and relieves PMS
- Helps normalize urine pH, relieving frequent urge to urinate
- Helps digestion, assimilation and balances the pH
- Helps relieve sore throats, laryngitis and throat tickles and cleans out throat and gum toxins
- Helps detox the body so sinus, asthma and flu sufferers can breathe easier and more normally
- Helps banish acne, athlete's foot, soothes burns, sunburns
- Helps prevent itching scalp, baldness, dry hair and banishes dandruff, rashes and shingles
- Helps fight arthritis and removes crystals and toxins from joints, tissues, organs and entire body
- Helps control and normalize body weight

– Paul C. Bragg, N.D., Ph.D. Health Crusader,
Originator of Health Food Stores

– 3 John 2 –

Our sincere blessings to you, dear friends, who make our lives so worthwhile and fulfilled by reading our teachings on natural living as our Creator laid down for us to follow. He wants us to follow the simple path of natural living. This is what we teach in our books and health crusades worldwide. Our prayers reach out to you and your loved ones for the best in health and happiness. We must follow the laws He has laid down for us, so we can reap this precious health physically, mentally, emotionally and spiritually!

HAVE AN APPLE HEALTHY LIFE!

With Love, Patricia Bragg

Braggs Organic Raw Apple Cider Vinegar with the "Mother Enzyme" is the #1 food I recommend to maintain the body's vital acid – alkaline balance.
–Gabriel Cousins, M.D., Author of *Conscious Eating*

Body Signs of Potassium Deficiency

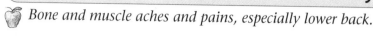

🍎 *Bone and muscle aches and pains, especially lower back.*

🍎 *The body feels heavy, tired and takes effort to move.*

🍎 *Shooting pains when straightening up after leaning over.*

🍎 *Dizziness upon straightening up after leaning over.*

🍎 *Morning dull headaches upon arising and when stressed.*

🍎 *Dull, faded-looking hair that lacks sheen and luster.*

🍎 *The scalp is itchy and dry. Dandruff and some premature hair thinning or balding may occur.*

🍎 *The hair is unmanageable, mats and often looks straw–like, and is sometimes extremely dry and other times oily.*

🍎 *The eyes itch, feel sore and uncomfortable and appear bloodshot and watery. Also, eyelids may be granulated with white matter.*

🍎 *The eyes tire easily and will not focus as they should.*

🍎 *You tire physically and mentally with the slightest effort.*

🍎 *Loss of mental alertness and onset of confusion, making decisions difficult. The memory fails, making you forget familiar names and places you should easily remember.*

🍎 *You become easily irritable and impatient with family, friends and loved ones and even with your business and social acquaintances.*

🍎 *You feel nervous, depressed, in a mental fog, and have difficulty getting things done due to mental and muscle fatigue. Even the slightest effort can leave you exhausted, upset and trembling.*

🍎 *At times, your hands and feet get chilled, even in warm weather.*

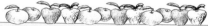

Potassium deficiency is a proven contributing cause of many illnesses, including: Arthritis, kidney stones, atrial fibrillation, adrenal insufficiency, celiac disease, high blood pressure, coronary artery disease, ulcerative colitis, hypothyroidism, irritable bowel syndrome, Alzheimer's disease, multiple sclerosis, myasthenia gravis, Crohn's disease, lupus, atherosclerosis, diabetes and stroke.
– Linda Page, N.D., Ph.D. **Healthy Healing** (visit her website: www.healthyhealing.com)

Pure Water is Important for Health

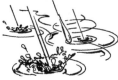

To the days of the aged it addeth length;
To the might of the strong it addeth strength;
It freshens the heart, it brings us delight;
It's like drinking a goblet of morning light.

The body is 70% water and purified or steam-distilled (chemical-free) water is important for total health. You should drink 7-9 glasses of water a day. Read our book, *Water – The Shocking Truth That Can Save Your Life* for more info on importance of pure water. See back pages for booklist.

Pure distilled water is important (page 42) in following The Bragg Healthy Lifestyle. Water is the key to all body functions including: digestion, circulation, bones and joints, assimilation, elimination, muscles, nerves, glands and senses. The right kind of water is one of your best natural protections against all kinds of diseases and viral infections, such as influenza and pneumonia. It is a vital factor in all body fluids, tissues, cells, lymph, blood and all glandular secretions. Water holds all nutritive factors in solution, as well as toxins and body wastes. It acts as the main transportation medium throughout the body, for both nutrition and cleansing detox purposes!

Low Fat Meals Cut Heart Disease Risk

A British research report by Dr. George Miller of Britain's Medical Research Council stated: *"High fat meals make the blood more prone to clot within 6 to 7 hours after eating. Low fat meals can almost immediately reverse this condition. Most heart attacks occur in the early morning. One reason may be the overnight clotting effects of a high fat dinner. Researchers feel that by cutting animal fats from your diet, you may be able to add years to your life and cut the risk of heart disease!"* Also recent research findings from Yale, Stanford, Harvard, University of California and the University of Chicago support Dr. Miller's 1993 statement that the safest *heart-healthy* meals are the organic plant based, low-fat, vegetarian diets with ample fruits and vegetables.

Dr. Dean Ornish has been able to reverse heart disease in more than 70% of his patients who follow, among other things, a low-fat vegetarian diet.

HEALTHY HEART HABITS FOR A LONG, VITAL LIFE

Remember, *organic live foods make live people. You are what you eat, drink, breathe, think, say and do.* So eat a low-fat, low-sugar, high-fiber diet of organic whole grains, sprouts, fresh salads, organic greens, vegetables, fruits, raw seeds, nuts, fresh juices and chemical-free, purified or distilled water.

Earn your food with daily exercise; for regular exercise, walking, etc. improves your health, stamina, go-power, flexibility and endurance and helps open the cardiovascular system. Only 45 minutes a day truly can do miracles for your heart, arteries, mind, nerves, soul and body! You become revitalized with new zest for living to accomplish your life goals!

We are made of tubes. To help keep them open, clean and to maintain good elimination, add 1 Tbsp of psyllium husk powder daily – hour after dinner – to juices, herbal teas and even the Bragg Vinegar Drink. Another way to guard against clogged tubes daily is add 1 to 2 Tbsps soy lecithin granules (*fat emulsifier-melts like butter*) over potatoes, veggies, soups and to juices, etc. Also take one cayenne capsule (40,000 HU) daily with a meal. Take 50 to 100 mgs regular-released niacin (B-3) with one meal daily to help cleanse and open the cardiovascular system, also improves memory. Skin flushing may occur; don't worry about this as it shows it's working! After cholesterol level reaches 180 then only take niacin twice weekly. Also studies show ½ tsp cinnamon powder is natures *statin* with no side effects.

The heart needs healthy balanced nutrients, so take natural multi-vitamin-mineral food supplements & extra heart helpers – mixed vitamin E, C, CoQ10, magnesium orotate, Omega-3, MSM, selenium, zinc, beta carotene & amino acids L-Carnitine, L-Taurine, L-Lysine & Proline. Folic acid, CoQ10, B6 & B12 helps keep homocysteine & CRP levels low. Hawthorn Berry extract brings relief for palpitations, arrhythmia, senile hearts and coronary disease. Take bromelain (from pineapple) and a multi-digestive enzyme with meals – aids and improves digestion, assimilation and elimination.

For sleep problems try 5-HTP tryptophan (an amino acid), melatonin, calcium, magnesium, valerian in caps, extract or tea, Bragg vinegar drink, chamomile or sleepytime herbal tea. For arthritis, osteoarthritis, pain/stiffness, try aloe gel or juice, glucosamine, chondroitin & MSM combo (caps, liquid & rollon), helps heal & regenerate. Also capsaicin & DMSO lotion helps heal.

Use amazing antioxidants – natural vitamin mixed E, C, Quercetin, grapeseed and grapefruit extract, CoQ10, selenium, SOD, etc. They improve immune system and help flush out dangerous free radicals that cause havoc with cardiovascular pipes and health. Research shows that antioxidants and enzymes promote longevity, slows ageing, fights toxins and cancer and helps prevent disease, cancer, cataracts, jet lag and exhaustion.

Recommended Blood Chemistry Values

- **Homocysteine:** 6 - 8 mcm/L – & **CRP (C-reactive protein high sensitivity):** lower than 1 mg/L low risk, 1-3 mg/L average risk, over 3 mg/L high risk
- **Total Cholesterol: Adults,** 180 mg/dl or less; 150 mg/dl is optimal **Children,** 140 mg/dl or less
- **HDL Cholesterol:** Men, 50 mg/dl or more; Women, 65 mg/dl or more
- **HDL Cholesterol Ratio:** 3.2 or less • **Triglycerides:** 100 mg/dl or less
- **LDL Cholesterol:** 100 mg/dl or less is optimal • **Glucose:** 80-100 mg/dl

Almost every known food may cause some allergic reaction at times. Thus, foods used in *elimination* diets may cause allergic reactions in some individuals. Some are listed among the *Most Common Food Allergies*. Since reaction to these foods is generally low, they are widely used in making test diets. By keeping a food journal and tracking your pulse rate after meals you will soon know your *problem* foods. Allergic foods cause pulse to go up. (Take base pulse before meals and then 30 minutes after meals. If it increases 8 -10 beats per minute – check foods for allergies.)

See web *http://members.aol.com/SynergyHN/allergy22b.html*

If your body has a reaction after eating some particular food, especially if it happens each time you eat that food, you may have an allergy. Some allergic reactions are: wheezing, sneezing, stuffy nose, nasal drip or mucus, dark circles, eye watering or waterbags under eyes, headaches, feeling light-headed or dizzy, fast heart beat, stomach or chest pains, diarrhea, extreme thirst, breaking out in a rash, swelling of extremities or stomach bloating, etc. (Do read Dr. Arthur Coca's book, *The Pulse Test – available from: amazon.com*)

If you know what you're allergic to, you are lucky; if you don't, you had better find out as fast as possible and eliminate all irritating foods from your diet. To re-evaluate your daily life and have a health guide to your future, start a daily journal (8½ x 11 notebook pg.145) of foods eaten, your pulse rate after meals and your reactions, moods, energy levels (ups & downs), weight, elimination and sleep patterns. You will soon discover the foods, situations, etc. causing problems. By charting your diet you will be amazed at the effects of eating certain foods. Paul Bragg faithfully kept a daily health journal for over 70 years.

If you are hypersensitive to certain foods, you must omit them from your diet! There are hundreds of allergies and of course it's impossible here to take up each one. Many have allergies to milk, wheat, or some are allergic to all grains. *Visit web: foodallergy.org.* Your daily health journal will help you discover and accurately pinpoint the foods and situations causing you problems. Start your health journal today!

Most Common Food Allergies

- *MILK: Butter, Cheese, Cottage Cheese, Ice Cream, Milk, Yogurt, etc.*
- *CEREALS & GRAINS: Wheat, Corn, Buckwheat, Oats, Rye*
- *EGGS: Cakes, Custards, Dressings, Mayonnaise, Noodles*
- *FISH: Shellfish, Crabs, Lobster, Shrimp, Shadroe*
- *MEATS: Bacon, Beef, Chicken, Pork, Sausage, Veal, Smoked Products*
- *FRUITS: Citrus Fruits, Melons, Strawberries*
- *NUTS: Peanuts, Pecans, Walnuts, chemically dried preserved nuts*
- *MISCELLANEOUS: Chocolate, Black Tea, Cocoa, Coffee, MSG, Palm and Cottonseed Oils, Salt, Spices and allergic reactions often caused by toxic pesticides on salad greens, vegetables, fruits, etc.*

Ten Common Sense Reasons Why You Should Only Drink Purified or Distilled Water!

- There are over 12,000 toxic chemicals on the market today and 500 more are being added yearly! Wherever you live, in the city or on a farm, some chemicals are getting into your drinking water. Beware chemicalized and fluorinated water.

- No one on the face of the earth today knows what effect these chemicals could have upon the body as they blend into thousands of different combinations. It is like making a mixture of colors; one drop could change the color.

- Proper equipment hasn't been designed yet to detect some of these chemicals and may not be for many years to come.

- The body is made up of 70% water, therefore, don't you think you should be particular about the type of water you drink? See important web: *www.Keepers-of-the-Well.org*

- The Navy has been drinking distilled water for years!

- Distilled water is chemical and mineral free. Distillation removes all chemicals and impurities possible from water.

- The body does need minerals . . . but it is not necessary that they come from water. There is not one mineral in water which cannot be found more abundantly in food! Water is the most unreliable source of minerals because it varies from one area to another. The food we eat – not the water we drink – is the best source of organic minerals!

- Distilled water is used for intravenous feeding, inhalation therapy, prescriptions and baby formulas. Therefore, doesn't it make common sense that it is good for everyone?

- Thousands of water distillers have been sold throughout the United States and around the world to individuals, families, dentists, doctors, hospitals, nursing homes and government agencies. All these informed and alert consumers are helping protect their health by using only steam distilled water. They don't want toxic chemicals!!

- With chemicals, pollutants and impurities in our water, it makes good sense to clean up the water you drink, by using Mother Nature's inexpensive way – distillation.

Pure water is the essential fluid of all life . . . the solvent of our ills and can be the deliverer of a radiant, healthy, long life. – Paul C. Bragg

One solution to America's soaring health costs is pure distilled water.

42

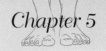

Chapter 5

Exercise Your Feet and Body

The Importance of Exercise

If we are to be free from foot injuries of all kinds, regardless of our age, we must keep them strong and sturdy with exercises! The muscles, bones and tendons all need vigorous exercise to give them the great power to withstand the strain we put upon them. A regular foot program should be followed daily, with sufficient time to be devoted to your precious, priceless feet.

There is one fact almost universally overlooked, the feet are encased in shoes for about 12 hours a day. In this time, their activity is limited and the full freedom for normal exercising of the tissues, muscles and tendons is inhibited. During most remaining hours, the feet are inactive in bed asleep. *(For foot comfort use pillows to elevate blankets to prevent drop foot problem)* Thus, for almost the full 24 hours, the feet get very little wholesome exercise, fresh air and sunshine (vitamin D) and are restricted and limited in normal functions. Their lack of activity offers a sharp contrast to the vigorous and constant foot-movements of shoeless natives in tropical warm climates.

Treatments for tired feet are all very well, but obviously it would be far better to avoid tired feet altogether. You can help in this respect with exercises to strengthen your feet. The stronger, more supple they are (with increased blood circulation activity), the less you will want to collapse at the end of a hard day.

Exercises for Healthy Feet and Toes

Here are some easy-to-do foot strengtheners. Learn what they are designed to do and how they are done. Do these exercises in your bare feet. Have absolutely no foot coverings, not even thin hosiery.

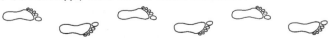

43

Make your two feet your best friends. – J. M. Barrie

Healthy Foot and Toe Exercises

Exercise No. 1

Stand with feet parallel, toes straight ahead, rise up on toes, then slowly come down. Do this about 20 times. This is best warm-up exercise for muscles and tendons of your feet.

Exercise No. 2

While seated, shoes and hosiery off, try picking up children's marbles, or something similar, with your toes. Don't use the same set of toes each time. Pick up the marbles with toes of one foot, let them drop to the floor, then try it with toes of the other foot. Do this for 5 minutes daily. It's fun. At first, you may find it difficult to grasp the marbles, etc. with toes, but after a few tries it becomes easier! All of the long tendons attached to the toes are strengthened by this exercise, and toes acquire more power to grip the ground and balance the feet.

Exercise No. 3

Stand barefoot on a thick, wide book so that the toes overlap the edge of the book. Move the toes over the edge of the book and grip. This should be done for several minutes each day. With each successive day the toes will show increased agility, and they will eventually be able to bend straight down, while the rest of the foot is horizontal. This strengthens the important toe tendons.

Exercise No. 4

While seated, place a pencil between your toes and try to write a letter. If this exercise is practiced for awhile, a legible letter may eventually be written. This uses the whole muscular structure of the foot, as well as the toes.

Exercise No. 5

While seated, firmly hold foot with one hand. With your other hand, take your big toe and rotate it around firmly, first one direction and then the other, then gently pull each toe. Now repeat this exercise on all toes. This keeps toes limber and helps reduce any (big toe) bunions.

Little things are like weeds – the longer we neglect them, the larger they grow.

It's strange that some men will drink and eat anything put before them, but will check very carefully the oil they put in their car.

Rolling Pin Foot Exercises

This is a great exercise for the feet. Use a rolling pin, either plain or model specifically for foot therapy with knobs. The latter is wonderful for reaching the reflex points of the feet, (page 118). Keep the rolling pin in living room so it will always be handy to use when watching TV.

Exercise No. 1

While seated, roll the pin from the toes to the heel, putting all the pressure you can take on the entire soles on the right foot and the left foot at the same time.

Exercise No. 2

Now stand and roll the pin from toes to heel, putting all the pressure you can first with one foot, then the other. This is an excellent exercise for building new feet from old. Every muscle, every bone, every nerve and tendon of the foot is ironed into its proper place. Spend plenty of time rolling the pin under the arches. You will feel the tiny crystals that may have formed, but with regular foot exercises, massage, reflexology and proper nutrition, these may soon disappear. These rolling pin exercises will pay you great dividends in foot health.

Vigorous Foot Walking Exercises

After a workout on the feet with the rolling pin, you are now ready to give the foot muscles, bones, nerves and tendons a workout for 10 minute sessions.

- Walk around on the **outer edges** of the feet.
- Walk around on the **inner edges** of the feet.
- Walk around just on **your heels.**
- Walk around just on **tiptoes.**

Walking this way may seem awkward, but these exercises will help strengthen and improve your feet.

Over 55% of Californians Overweight: *Despite the healthy tofu-and-avocado image Californians enjoy across the U.S., over half the state's adults and even the children are overweight. Researchers interviewed 4,149 people in all (1,772 men, 2,377 women) by telephone recently and found that 55% were overweight or obese! This is the latest study in 10 years. Even back in 1990, 44.6% of Californians were overweight or obese.* – News Service Report

---

When recovering from accidents, fractures, etc. take extra natural, mineral and vitamin supplements to nourish and help your body heal faster.

Enjoy Barefoot Ground Contact Exercises

When possible walk barefoot on your grass, lawn (or local parks,etc.), as often as possible. *Caution: Check and avoid golf course toxic lawns, and any that use toxins on grass.*

If you can walk on a sandy beach you are giving the feet the greatest of all tonics! When you walk on the beach your feet are walking naturally. Every part of the foot is activated as it should be. We have seen people with the most crippled and battered feet spend several months or more at a beach and emerge with whole new feet! Whether it be in Florida, California, Hawaii, or any other sandy spot, walking on the sand will do as much for your heart and soul as it will for your feet. With its uneven, undulating surface, its deep drifts that become smooth at the water's edge, the beach is an ideal place to walk that gives your entire foot a massage with each step!

Learn Lessons from Mother Nature

Walking on the lawn or sand is the finest of all foot exercises! It acts as a stimulant to all the foot tissues. A child's ordinary sandbox or even smooth, small "pea" gravel in a box is ideal for this exercise. The sand or gravel fits the contours of the sole and the arch, acting as a healthy foot and ankle stimulator at the same time.

The most significant points to remember about foot exercising are: (1) at least one-half hour daily must be devoted to foot improvement, and (2) the exercises must be followed with faithful regularity. Only under these conditions, plus your healthy nutritional diet and foot therapy schedule, will any gratifying results be realized!

Your Dynamic Foot Springiness Plan

No matter how you have abused your feet in the past, the foot program will help you! Carry a picture in your mind of the kind of feet you wish to mold through this health foot program. Let nothing stop you as you work on your schedule for attaining healthier, stronger feet that are going to carry you through your entire life!

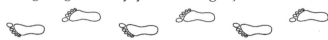

46

Use your willpower and better judgement to select and eat only the foods which are best for you, regardless of any ridicule or gibes of friends. – Dr. Richard T. Field

Walking Promotes Healthy Feet

There is nothing as pleasurable as walking, it's the most ideal exercise in the world (*See Chapter 9, page 97*). When taking a walk, open wide your eyes, mind, heart and soul to discover the miracles around you! You will see new beauty in trees, blooming flowers, singing birds, etc. The Seasons of Mother Nature are so rewarding to watch, because each has its own individual beauty!

If you have *feet that are killing you*, all these joys of walking are gone. Many people forego the pleasure of walking because their feet cry out in pain with every step. So, use this Bragg Foot Culture Program to find new joy in taking healthy walks. Dancing is also a pleasure we enjoy and can be a pain-free joy. There is nothing that can relax us more and give us the abandoned joy of living as dancing does. But, like walking for pleasure, dancing requires strong, happy feet! These great pleasures in life require painfree, ageless, healthy feet. You can win back youthful feeling feet by being determined to never miss a day in following this foot care program.

Prove it to Yourself – You Can Have Healthy Feet

Day by day, by faithfully following this Natural Bragg Foot Culture Program, you will see wonderful changes in your feet. They will feel as though they belong to a barefoot, strong and sturdy carefree child, of which you will be proud. They will be supple, flexible and free from pain. You will regain the feeling of springiness in your new feet. Is this worth working for? Just how important are your feet to you? Remember they must carry you through life! So you should treat them with your full respect, so that they can be your constant companion of delight and joy with every step you take!

Websites to inspire you to enjoy Healthy Walking and Hiking Programs in your area:

- *www.justwalk.com* • *www.gorp.com/gorp/activity/hiking.htm*
- *www.fitconnection.com* • *www.activevideos.com/walking.htm*
- *www.outdoorsclub.org/index1.htm* • *www.sierraclub.com*

The average man walks 7 miles a day and the average woman walks 10.
– American College of Foot & Ankle Surgeons

KEEP HEALTHY & YOUTHFUL BIOLOGICALLY WITH EXERCISE & GOOD NUTRITION

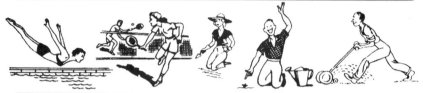

Always remember you have the following important reasons for following The Bragg Healthy Lifestyle:

- The ironclad laws of Mother Nature and God.
- Your common sense, which tells you that you are doing right.
- Your aim to make your health better and your life longer.
- Your resolve to prevent illness so that you may enjoy life.
- Make an art of healthy living; you will be youthful at any age.
- You will retain your faculties and be hale, hearty, active and useful far beyond the ordinary length of years.
- You will possess more super mental and physical powers!

WANTED – For Robbing Health & Life

KILLER Saturated Fats	CHOKER Hydrogenated Fats
CLOGGER Salt	DEADEYED Devitalized Foods
DOPEY Caffeine	HARD WATER Inorganic Minerals
PLUGGER Frying Pan	FLUORIDE Health Distroyer
DEATH-DEALER Drugs	CRAZY Alcohol
GREASY Overweight	SMOKY Tobacco
HOGGY Overeating	LOAFER Laziness

What Wise Men Say

Wisdom does not show itself so much in precept as in life – a firmness of mind and mastery of the appetite. – Seneca

I saw few die of hunger – of eating, a hundred thousand.
– Ben Franklin

Govern well thy appetite, lest Sin surprise thee, and her black attendant, Death. – Milton

Your health is your wealth.
– Paul C. Bragg

Our prayers should be for a sound mind in a healthy body. – Juvenal

Health is a blessing that money cannot buy. – Izaak Walton

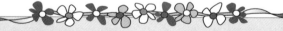

48

The natural healing force within us is the greatest force in getting well.
– Hippocrates, Father of Medicine, 400 BC

Of all the knowledge, the one most worth having is knowledge about health! The first requisite of a good life is to be a healthy person. – Herbert Spencer

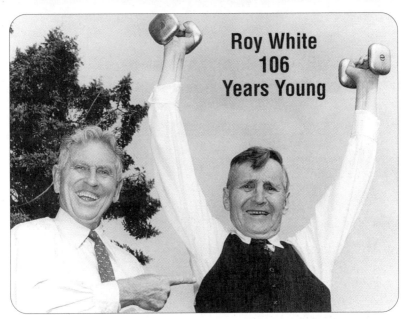

**Roy White
106
Years Young**

Paul C. Bragg and Roy White
Bragg's Weight Lifting Health Follower

My father's good friend, Roy White of Long Beach, California, is in his 106th year of life, yet he has a tireless, painless and ageless body. He knows the Laws of Mother Nature and God and he lives by them. He doesn't fear old age and is a young man in biological years. We both could name many, many more friends who are in their 80s, 90s and even over 100, who are biologically youthful!

Iron Pumping Oldsters (86 to 96) Triple Their Muscle Strength in U.S. Study

WASHINGTON – Ageing nursing home residents in Boston study "pumping iron"? Elderly weightlifters tripling and quadrupling their muscle strength? Is it possible? Most people would doubt and wonder! Government experts on ageing answered those questions with a resounding "yes" with the results of this revealing and amazing study! They turned a group of frail Boston nursing home residents, aged 86 to 96, into weightlifters to demonstrate that it's never too late to reverse age-related declines in muscle strength. The group participated in a regimen of high-intensity weight-training in a study conducted by Dr. Maria A. Fiatarone of the Agriculture Department's Human Nutrition Research Center on Ageing at Tufts University in Boston.

Visit interesting web: www2.fhs.usyd.edu.au/ess/fiatarone

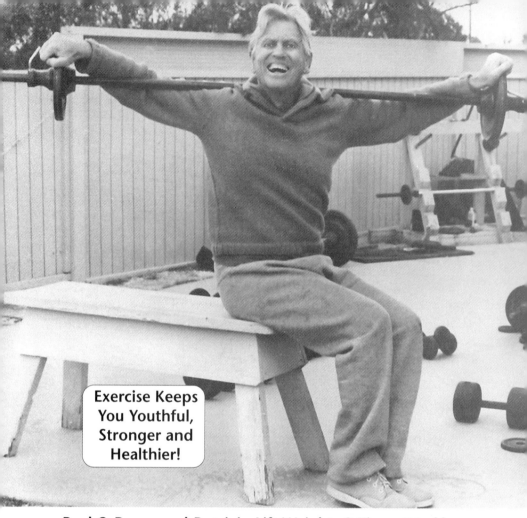

Exercise Keeps You Youthful, Stronger and Healthier!

Paul C. Bragg and Patricia Lift Weights 3 Times Weekly

A few of the participants did report minor muscle and joint aches, but 9 of the 10 completed the program. One man, aged 86, felt a pulling sensation at the site of a previous hernia incision and dropped out after 4 weeks.

The study participants, drawn from a 712 bed long-term care facility in Boston, worked out 3 times a week. They performed 3 sets of 8 repetitions with each leg on a weight-lifting machine. The weights were gradually increased from about 10 pounds initially, to about 40 pounds at the end of the eight week program. Fiatarone said the study carries some strong important health implications to improve the wellness and fitness of older people, who represent a growing proportion of the U.S. population. A decline in muscle strength, tone and muscle size is the more predictable feature of ageing.

Amazing Strength Results in 8 Weeks

"The favorable response to strength training in our subjects was remarkable in light of their very advanced ages, extremely sedentary habits, multiple chronic diseases, functional disabilities and also nutritional inadequacies. The elderly weight-lifters increased their muscle strength by anywhere from three-fold to four-fold in as little as eight weeks." Fiatarone said they probably were stronger at the end of the program than they had been in years! Fiatarone and her associates emphasized the safety of such a closely supervised weight-lifting program, even among people in frail health. The average age of the 10 elderly participants, for instance, was 90. Six had coronary heart disease; seven had arthritis; six had bone fractures resulting from osteoporosis; four had high blood pressure; and all had been physically inactive for years. Yet, no serious medical problems resulted from the program, only good results!

Muscle strength in the average adult decreases by 30% to 50% during the course of life. Some experts on ageing do not know whether the decrease is an unavoidable consequence of ageing or results mainly from sedentary lifestyle and other controllable factors.

Muscle atrophy and weakness are not merely cosmetic problems in elderly people, but huge health problems, especially with the frail elderly! Researchers linked muscle weakness with recurrent falls, a major cause of immobility and death among the elderly population. This causes millions yearly in staggering medical costs.

Previous studies have suggested that weight-training can be helpful in reversing age-related muscle weakness! Dr. Fiatarone said physicians have been reluctant to recommend weightlifting for frail elderly with multiple health problems. This government study might be changing their minds for it shows the great importance of keeping the 640 muscles as active and fit as possible to maintain general good health for all ages!

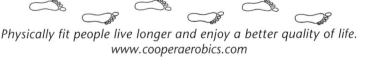

Physically fit people live longer and enjoy a better quality of life.
www.cooperaerobics.com

The chemistry of the food a person eats becomes his own body chemistry.

Food for Thought

The body and the mind are so closely connected that not even a single word, thought or action can come into existence without being reflected in the personality and the health of the individual. – John Prentiss

---

If you want permanent change, you have to change permanently.
– Dan Robey, Author, The Power of Positive Thoughts, a Bragg Follower
www.thepowerofpositivehabits.com

When you live The Bragg Healthy Lifestyle you can help activate your own powerful internal defense arsenal and maintain it at top efficiency. However, if you continue unhealthy eating habits, it's harder for your body to fight off illness! – Paul C. Bragg, N.D.,Ph.D.

Nutrition directly affects growth, development, repreduction, well-being of an individual's physical and mental condition. Health depends upon nutrition more than on any other single factor – Dr. Wm. H, Sebrell, Jr.

A reminder: What's on the plate, becomes what's on the chair.

Everything is brighter in the new dawn's light –
especially after a recharging good night's sleep!

Perhaps the most valuable result of all: a wise, good education is the ability to make yourself do the right thing, when it ought to be done, as it should be done, whether you like to do it or not!

Staying in shape pays, partly because aerobic activity promotes circulation. If you already have back problems, the right kind of regular exercise will help prevent you from getting more severe pain and further injury.
– Stephen Hochschuler, M.D., orthopedic surgeon and chariman,
Texas Back Institute, Plano, Texas.

Shocking Fact: 25% of hospital deaths are due to medical doctor errors. Play it safe – before any prescriptions, chemical drug treatments (chemo, etc.) or serious surgery, it's best to get 2 to 3 evaluations to be positive you are making the right decision for your future health! Once treatment or surgery is done, it is often too late to make amends, so the time to get consultation is before, not after the fact! It's your body and your right to help and judge in all decisions of your health and future well-being! See web: www.doctormalpractice.info

England's Oldest Champion Runner

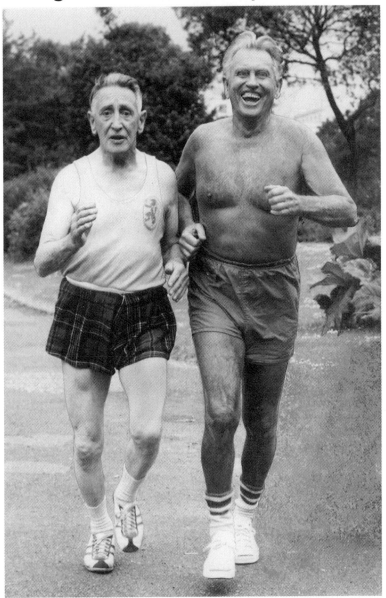

Duncan McLean and Paul C. Bragg in London

Duncan McLean, England's oldest Champion Sprinter (93 years young), on a training run with Paul C. Bragg in London's famous Regent's Park. They both have enjoyed a healthy lifetime with strong, active, ageless feet.

People who follow healthy living habits in early adulthood spend less time coping with disability and illness in their later years. – Stanford University

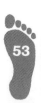

You will increase your health, joy, energy, peace of mind and improve sleep with more daily exercise and deep breathing.

Exercise and Eat for Total Health

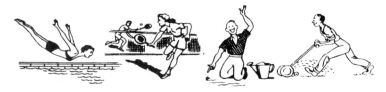

Enjoy Bragg Healthy Lifestyle
For a Lifetime of Super Health

In a broad sense, "The Bragg Healthy Lifestyle for the Total Person" is a combination of physical, mental, emotional, social and spiritual components. The ability of the individual to function effectively in his environment depends on how smoothly these components function as a whole. Of all the qualities that comprise an integrated personality, a totally healthy, fit body is one of the most desirable . . . so start today to achieve your health goals!

A person may be said to be totally physically fit if he functions as a total personality with efficiency and without pain or discomfort of any kind. This is to have a Painless, Tireless, Ageless body. One possessing sufficient muscular strength and endurance to maintain a healthy posture and successfully carry on the duties imposed by life and the environment. To be able to handle emergencies and have enough energy for recreation and social obligations after the "work day" has ended. It is to meet the requirements of his environment through possessing the resilience to recover rapidly from fatigue, tension, stress and strain of daily living without the aid of stimulants, drugs or alcohol. To be able to enjoy natural recharging sleep at night and awaken fit and alert in the morning for the challenges of the new fresh day ahead.

Keeping the body totally healthy and fit is not a job for the uninformed or the careless person. It requires an understanding of the body and of a healthy lifestyle and then following it for a long, happy lifetime of health! The result of "The Bragg Healthy Lifestyle" is to wake up the possibilities within you, rejuvenate your body, mind and soul to total balanced health. It's within your reach, so don't procrastinate, start today! Our hearts go out to touch your heart with nourishing, caring love for your total health and life!

Patricia Bragg and *Paul C. Bragg*

54

Dear friend, I wish above all things that thou may prosper and be in health even as the soul prospers. – 3 John 2

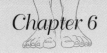

Chapter 6

Foot Care for Life

Foot Care During Pregnancy

Because of weight gain and postural changes during pregnancy, foot and leg fatigue can become pronounced. There may be tiredness and heaviness, leg cramping and even the development of varicose veins. In most cases, these symptoms will disappear after the baby is born. In any case, proper foot care during pregnancy is important for the health of both mother and child.

Wearing comfortable shoes to support you is vital. These should have the lowest and broadest heel that feels good. Since your feet might swell, especially in hot weather, the shoe must be large and flexible enough to allow for changes in foot size. There should be no hard pressure on the top of the foot or on the toes.

Don't wear shoes made of plastic, patent leather or synthetics that aren't flexible, and *will not give* with your foot. Your shoes should allow your feet to be flexible and breathe. The soles and heels are especially important. They should provide adequate support and cushioning without jarring or binding you. Flexible rubber or crepe soles, which are firm, yet springy, are generally better than hard leather bottoms. Women are best to avoid high heels, since pregnancy already changes your posture, why do further damage by misaligning yourself?

Your socks and hose should be large enough to allow free toe movement. If you are advised to wear *support* hosiery, don't wear the tight advertised elastic hose - they cause undue compression of the feet and legs. Instead, buy toeless (and sometimes heelless) seamless surgical hosiery and you can wear your usual hose or socks over them. Be careful that your socks do not have tight elastic bands which interfere with blood flow and can increase swelling.

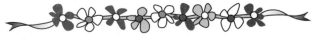

Babies and giving birth are blessings and miracles of life. – Patricia Bragg

Elevate, Exercise and Rest Your Feet

Raising and resting your feet on a pillow at night for sleeping, during a noon nap or when watching TV in the evening can help cut down swelling and cramping. While your feet are elevated, try flexing them, gripping with your toes, then curling them back, rotating your feet both ways at the ankles, and any other movements which increase your circulation and ease of motion. Follow the Bragg Foot Program and do the foot and walking exercises and faithfully follow The Bragg Health Lifestyle and healthy diet, plus go barefoot whenever possible. Give yourself and your baby the best possible first steps into their new healthy life! Remember, babies are blessed miracles!

Caring for Children's Feet from Birth

When the fetus is only six weeks old, the feet and legs have already begun to develop. At birth, the average infant's foot length is slightly a little over three inches. Eventually, the feet will grow to about 8 inches (average) in length for women, and about 11 inches in length for a man. To promote proper foot development, the baby's feet should be monitored and attended to carefully.

Barefoot is best, especially for babies! The bones in their little feet are still soft and not yet fully formed. Why compress them with shoes? Give their bare feet a chance to move, wiggle, stretch and grow without any restriction. Don't constrict circulation and motion of the baby's developing, growing feet with *prison-like* shoes! Foot exercise is very important when you are pregnant.

The only reason to cover your infant's feet is to keep them warm. To do so, use non-stretch socks of natural fabric, or a baby garment with feet and legs, as long as the garment is not too tight. Check for shrinkage after washing and be sure baby hasn't outgrown it. When covering the infant with a blanket, don't tuck it in tightly. Either tuck loosely or allow the blanket to simply rest on the feet and legs. Free movement is the key.

A strong body makes a strong mind. –Thomas Jefferson, 3rd U.S. President, 1801-1809

Your Baby Needs Love and Massages

Baby's position in the crib is also important. Don't let your baby always lie on their stomach. Turn the baby at intervals while he or she is sleeping. This helps promote balanced muscular development and prevents problems such as toenails which are curved in toward the toes due to a constant on-the-belly resting position.

When diapering your child, notice whether the feet, legs, and bottom are symmetrical. If you see any difference between the two sides, consult your doctor. Also, do not diaper baby with bulky diapers. These force the legs into an unnatural, outward position. Fortunately, new diaper materials are generally thin enough to prevent this problem. Before or after diapering, gently massage your baby's feet, spine, and entire body when time allows to promote nerve development and healthy circulation. Remember foot and body massages are good for all ages!

Do not dangle your baby to get him or her to walk faster. This puts strain on the arms, neck, spine and entire system. Respect Mother Nature's timetable; your child will stand and walk only when the foot and leg muscles are ready to support and move the entire body. Generally, an infant will attempt to crawl at about six months, try to stand at eight, will be able to stand well at about 12 months, and will walk unaided at 14 months or more. These are averages and have nothing to do with your child's ultimate coordination. In Mother Nature, each child develops at its own rate. Don't let misguided parental pride interfere with the natural course of things!

The Feet of Youth

It has been estimated that one-third of young children in this country have abnormal foot posture. This means that one out of every three people growing up in America is presently headed for aches, pains and worse throughout the years due to the fact that no one took the time or trouble to examine, care for and if necessary, correct the youth's foot problems. It is true that almost all of us are born with perfect feet and that, naturally, the foot will develop well. But parents must examine their children's feet and encourage proper foot care habits in order to give them a good start on the path of healthy feet for life!

When your youngster begins to get up on his or her feet in the playpen, put a blanket or soft rug over the mattress. This will allow your child to begin to grip with the toes and to stand on a soft, yet firm surface. When he or she begins to walk, don't worry about awkwardness of movement or the lack of an arch on the foot. Unless a baby is exceptionally thin, there is a fatty pad under the arch which won't disappear until two-and-a-half or three years of age, and then the arch starts to show.

Food For Thought

The first wealth is health. – Emerson

The US Congress should immediately ban all ads aimed at children that promote foods high in fat and sugar – these unhealthy, nutrient - poor, high - calorie foods become life-long eating habits that are potentially life-threatening! The Fast Foods Industry and their thousands of restaurants serve millions of meals daily that accelerate the growth of fast foods and have changed America's eating habits! Obesity is now epidemic! – Marion Nestle, Author of *Food Politics, How the Food Industry Influences Nutrition and Health. Web: www.ucpress.edu*

The nervousness and peevishness of our times are chiefly attributable to tea and coffee. The digestive organs of confirmed coffee drinkers are in a state of chronic derangement which reacts on the brain, producing fretful and lachrymose moods. – Dr. Bock, 1910

Sir Isaac Newton, when writing his great work, "Principia," lived wholly upon a vegetable diet.

The word "vegetarian" is not derived from "vegetable," but from the Latin, homo vegetus, among the Romans meaning a strong, robust, thoroughly healthy man.

The desire for salty foods is an acquired taste. Your tastebuds can be retrained to appreciate the true flavors of foods. – Neal Barnard, M.D., *Food for Life*

Prayer is the mortar that holds our house together. – Sister Teresa

Monitor Children's Feet and Their Walking and Choose Their Shoes Wisely

Unfortunately, one can't walk around the modern world barefoot forever! When it comes time to fit your child with shoes, use the same guidelines (see Chapter 8) that you use to select your own comfortable shoes.

It's important to consistently inspect the way your child walks when he begins to do so. The best time to examine your child's gait is when he is barefoot, not when wearing tight, non flexible shoes! Does the child toe-in or toe-out consistently? Is he or she knock-kneed or bow-legged to an unusual degree? Does your youngster limp consistently, or walk only on the toes or heels?

None of these conditions are necessarily cause for alarm, but all should be checked by a pediatrician, orthopedist or podiatrist and also a chiropractor! The condition may be transient and hopefully disappear by itself with your guidance. However, it may be caused by improper bone or muscle development, perhaps due to faulty nutrition or defective metabolic functioning, etc. Checking with an expert is the only way to be sure!

As you bathe and massage your child, examine their feet. Look especially for small growths. A corn, callus or wart may be an indication of an underlying condition which is correctable if caught early! Also inspect nails, especially if nail-biting is a problem. If the area around nails is tender due to tearing or biting, soaking feet in warm water (add 1 Tbsp. Bragg Organic Vinegar) or foot wrap for 10 to 15 minutes can help relieve pain and hasten healing. If nail-biting is severe, promptly consult their pediatrician.

Growing Pains - the cramps in legs some children get between 2 and 5 years old are no longer considered normal. There is a reason: poor posture, fatigue or faulty nutrition. Relief can be given by multiple vitamin and mineral supplements (especially calcium, magnesium and vitamin D), massaging, keeping bedroom temperature warm enough, and by making sure one leg doesn't continually rest on the other during sleep. If growing pains persist, please see your health practitioner.

59

Shoes Should Fit Right and Be Flexible

Children's shoes should be fitted so that when the child is standing, the shoe toe box is at least a half-inch longer than the longest toe (not necessarily the big toe). The shoe should not press down on the child's toes or on top of foot. The shoe should fit snug, but not tightly at the heel. The heel should be firmly cradled, not slip or wiggle in the shoe, this can cause painful blisters.

The shoe itself should be flexible, with a shock-absorbing sole and heel, and should allow the foot to breathe. Shoes which come high on the ankles are not necessary. Ankles must be allowed to strengthen to support the body weight and be allowed to develop flexibility. Under no circumstances should you cram your child's feet into stylish, grown-up shoes or boots such as miniature high heels or cowboy boots. Best to keep the shoe light, roomy and the sole flexible!

By the same token, do not buy shoes that are far too large for your youngster's foot on the theory that he or she will grow into them. How would you like to have to walk around in shoes two sizes too large and get blisters, calluses, etc., because your feet will someday enlarge with age? Buy your child shoes that fit correctly, right now! Beware of hand-me-downs and resoled shoes that don't fit well. If any foot or walking problem arises, see a foot doctor to get at the cause of the difficulty; don't just cover it up or try to force the foot to change.

When your child has worn his or her new shoes for a day or two, check the feet for signs of any irritations. Sometimes these can be avoided by working the shoe at a particular spot, or by changing or loosening the lacing pattern. If the irritation persists, change the shoes. Proper footwear does not require much breaking in, since it is often the foot that is being broken! Socks, too, should be checked to insure that they are not too small, haven't shrunk in the wash and do not bind the foot or restrict circulation. Remember, getting your child off on a good footing will pay dividends in ease, comfort and freedom of movement throughout their long, healthy, happy life!

115,000 Miles Walked in Average Lifetime

In your lifetime, you'll walk about 115,000 miles, about half the distance to the moon! Obviously, the condition of your feet will make all the difference in the world as to whether your steps are positive and productive, or painful and impoverished. It's up to you!

It is estimated that 80 percent of all adults suffer some form of foot problem, and surveys show most Americans believe it is normal for feet to hurt. Normal it is not! By following the Bragg Foot Culture Program, you can be one of the lucky, healthy, 20 percent of adults who stride through life freely, on happy, pain-free feet!

The adult foot is composed of 26 bones, 4 arches, 19 muscles, 33 joints, and 107 ligaments, all of which have to be strong and flexible enough to support the body through two-thirds of its passage on earth. When feet are in good working order, they send confident, stable messages to the brain via the nervous system. Sore feet only feed the brain messages of instability and pain.

Each step we take begins with the body weight being carried by the heel. The weight then shifts to the outside of the foot and, finally we push off with the ball of the foot and the big toe. The toes constantly serve to help maintain balance. The fatty pads on the bottom of the feet act as shock absorbers when the feet contact the ground.

Normally, all parts of the foot function well and work together to create stable support and locomotion. Barring major injury, they will continue to do so throughout life. However, there are a number of minor complaints and conditions that can slow you down unless you're aware of what they are and how to either prevent or heal them.

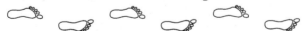

The average person takes approximately 8,000 steps per day.
– Dr. Jessica R. Luck, Podiatrist

The beautiful thing about learning is that
no one can take it away from you. – B.B. King

When you know what you want, and want it
badly enough, you will find a way to get it!

We have compiled a list of some of the most common foot problems and solutions. However, there are many remedies for foot ailments, based on different medical theories. It may take more additional research and some experimentation on your part to find the right solution for your particular foot problem. It is possible that the nature of your ailment will require you to treat it in ways other than the ones we have outlined here. As always, don't hesitate to seek a qualified foot doctor's opinion or to get a second or third opinion!

First, Check Your Overall Lifestyle and Habits

When you find yourself in need of treatment, there are a number of factors you must consider before embarking upon a particular course. Your overall lifestyle is one of the first things on the list. In most cases your diet, sleeping habits, physical and mental activities, hobbies, occupation and geographical climate will play a part in your general health or lack thereof. Also examine your mental, emotional and spiritual state of being as well. Know yourself! An honest appraisal of these factors will yield valuable info that will be very useful in determining the best way to treat any of your problems so you can plan, plot and take action to make yourself healthy! Please keep in mind that foot diseases and conditions, especially chronic ones, are just like any other type of malady in that they are usually a direct result of certain actions, activities and lifestyles. Because of this, some people will be more likely to develop specific foot problems than others. For example, people whose jobs require them to be on their feet all day, like teachers, clerks, dentists, doctors, nurses, and athletes, are more inclined to develop recurrent foot problems than people in more sedentary careers.

Healthy body, bones and feet come from healthy foods, habits and lifestyle.
– Patricia Bragg, N.D., Ph.D., Health Crusader

55% of Americans missed a day of work last year because of foot problems.
– American Podiatric Medical Association, www.apma.org

Former U.S. Surgeon General Koop warned Americans back in a 1988 report on Nutrition and Health that diet-related diseases account for 68% of deaths!

Self discipline is your golden key; without it, you can't be happy and healthy.
– Maxwell Maltz, M.D. author *Psycho-Cybernetics* and a Bragg follower

How to Treat Foot Blisters

Blisters are irritated areas which become very tender and filled with either air or fluid just under the skin. They are caused by part of an ill-fitting shoe rubbing against the affected area of the foot. They frequently occur when new shoes are worn and can be prevented by going barefoot when possible, wearing thick enough hose, or by flexing stiff areas of the shoe prior to wearing them. Remember, if a shoe requires much breaking in, it didn't fit right in the first place! Buy shoes cautiously!

In general, do not pop blisters. This can increase the irritation and sometimes promote infection. It's better to wait things out and keep the tender area protected when wearing shoes. Also exposure to air will speed healing blisters and let Mother Nature take its course.

Blisters can be avoided if you are sensitive enough to feel the affected area beginning to become irritated. Remove or change shoes, or at least cover affected area with a band-aid or a cushioning "second skin" product such as moleskin.

How to Treat Foot Calluses

Calluses are patches of rough, dry, dead and hardened skin that may form on the ball of the foot or on other flat areas. Calluses are caused by recurrent pressure or friction, usually produced by poorly fitted shoes, or by bad habits of walking and standing. These move the feet out of line with the shoe, or promote slipping or tilting of the shoe with respect to the foot. Again, the difficulty may be either with the shoes, a misaligned foot, or your posture.

If the shoes are causing calluses, either cushion the insides or buy new shoes. Calluses may be painful and get worse through continued irritation. If the problem, then is in the feet themselves, changing shoes will not be the total answer. What's necessary is following 100% the Bragg Foot Health Program faithfully, and also improving posture and walking strides. *More info page 79.*

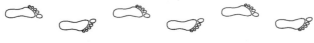

63

American health care costs are soaring up and up!!!

Immediate relief from a callus may be obtained by placing a thin piece of moleskin directly over callus, but separated from it by cotton or gauze. When you remove the moleskin each day, flex your foot to hold skin taut, then slowly pull the moleskin off. Never rip off covering, or you may end up with a bleeding callus!

Opinion is divided among experts whether to use a pumice stone or callus wand to file down a callus, *both are O.K.* Please be gentle and don't overdo and irritate area!!! Caution: *Feet do need some natural fat padding!*

How to Treat Foot Corns

Corns, like calluses, are caused by repeated rubbing or pressure on the skin. The irritation increases blood supply to the area and the cells grow in an accelerated fashion, causing a corn. Corns tend to occur on the toes: on top, on the sides, or between the toes. Since corns are cone-shaped, with the tip penetrating into the tender tissue underneath, they can be especially painful. Beware of over-the-counter medications which claim to remove the *root* of the problem, because corns have no root! Incidentally, many corn cure products contain an acid which eats away the corn and also surrounding healthy tissue and can cause ulcerations. Always use caution!

Soft corns are usually found between toes, often in pairs, facing one another. They are caused when the bones of the opposing toes rub against one another. Seed corns are small and often develop in groups. They are frequently found on the soles and may be a result of irritation from protruding shoe tacks. Sometimes a corn will develop within a callus, creating double trouble!

As with calluses, development of corns does not necessarily show that the fault is with the shoe. Your posture or gait may be pushing a perfectly good shoe out of shape and your aching foot with it. Do all your shoes produce irritation in the same places? If so, this is a fairly sure indication that you need to become more aware of your feet and their misalignment.

May you live healthy all the days of your life. – Jonathan Swift

If you want to use a corn pad to obtain immediate relief, make certain it doesn't contain an oval area with acid in it. If it does, cut out this oval area. You can make a horseshoe-shaped pad and stick it just behind and around the corn. The pad should not rub up against the corn, for that will just increase the irritation.

A better idea is to use a simple spot band-aid. Place the band-aid with the sterile gauze spot directly over the corn. If you have a soft corn on the toe, you can also wrap soft material such as lamb's wool around the toe. Don't wrap it too tight, as this restricts the circulation.

For both corns and calluses, remove any dressing and wash the area each evening. It's best to leave the area uncovered at night and allow Mother Nature to do her healing. Don't, under any circumstances use a razor blade to try to cut out the corn or callus. This will make things far worse. If the problem is that severe, consult your foot doctor! Remember, corns and calluses will disappear if you don't wear wrong-fitting tight shoes. Go barefoot as often as possible and your feet will thank you!

How to Treat Ingrown Toenails

Much confusion exists concerning ingrown toenails. The nails don't really *grow into* the flesh at either side. What happens is that the side flesh is forced into and over the sides of the nail. The cause is either undue pressure on the toes and nails or improper cutting of the nails.

If your shoes are too short or too tight, they may exert constant pressure on the toes, especially the big toe, causing ingrown toenails. To prevent this, make sure there is a half-inch of space between the longest toe and the front of the shoe, and that the toe box is not too narrow.

Proper cutting of the toenails is done straight across, without cutting down into the nail grooves. It used to be thought that ingrown toenails could be cured by cutting a wedge in the center of the nail, since the nail would then grow inward to fill the wedge. This is not true! The nail always grows straight out from the bottom, taking about 120 days to make the full trip out to cutting length.

If the ingrown toenail is not too severe, and if it is not infected, it may be treated by soaking the foot in warm vinegar water for 5-10 minutes several times a day. This greatly relieves irritation. Don't attempt to cut down into nail groove on either side to relieve pressure. If you do, you may leave small bony hooks or spicules on the nail that will cut into the flesh and cause painful, irritated flesh to form at the edge of the nail grooves. To relieve the soreness of the side grooves, gently work a little absorbent cotton between the nail and the flesh. If these measures do not give relief, or if other, more severe, nail problems develop, promptly see a podiatrist.

Other Common Foot Ailments

Plantar Warts - which may appear on the soles of feet, are caused by a virus and may be related to stress, which increases susceptibility to the virus. Warts can be contagious and frequently family members may develop them. If someone in your family has developed a wart or warts, make sure he or she has his own bath mat and towel, since wet, porous surfaces may contain the virus. The bathtub or the shower stall bottom itself, which is nonporous, will probably not harbor the virus. Adequate intake of Vitamin C and CoQ10 daily is important to maintain immunity against viruses that cause warts.

Warts - to remove try crushing garlic clove and apply directly to wart area only, or try caster oil or vinegar poultice and cover with bandage and leave on for 24 hours. Warts may disappear on their own. Don't attempt to burn or cut off warts yourself. If, after reasonable time, they don't disappear, see your foot doctor for treatment. Unless wart becomes bothersome, sore or interferes with walking, there is no need to see a doctor.

Heel Spurs may develop on the back of heels from continued shoe irritation or a foot injury. They are bony growths that require professional treatment. **Rashes** may be caused by a number of factors and are often allergy-related. **Excess Sweating** can be helped by detox diet and fasting. **Hammertoes** and bunions are ailments that

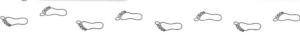

usually require medical attention. **Hammertoes** or toes that curve upward in the middle, can be made worse by shoes that are too short or tight. **Bunions,** buildup of bone at joint of foot where it meets the big toe, are caused by wrong shoes and can make walking painful. **Diabetics** who are prone to circulatory problems, should pay special attention to foot ailments and consult a doctor promptly if they arise! Also diabetics should not do *hot* foot soaks or *hot* baths. They can use vinegar and other herbal solutions in warm water soaks or gently sponged on.

All of the above difficulties are caused or made worse by irritation or unnatural restriction of the feet. By following the Bragg System of Natural Foot Culture, which involves healthy diet, hygiene and exercise, these common foot miseries can be curtailed or prevented!

The great thing in life is not so much where you stand, but in what direction you are moving.

Most Americans' bodies thirst for pure distilled water! Their bodies become sick, prematurely aged, crippled and stiff due to chemicalized water, inorganic minerals and lack of sufficient pure water (8 glasses daily)!

High homocysteine blood levels (safe – 6-8 mcm/L) & dietary deficiencies of vitamins (B12, folic acid and CoQ10) are underlying causes of heart, diabetes, osteoporosis and kidney diseases. – Kilmer S. McCully, M.D., Author of "The Homocysteine Revolution" available at Amazon.com Visit this informative web – www.homocysteine.com

Dr. Stephen T. Sinatra recommends CoQ10 supplements to combat heart disease, cancer, gum disease and ageing. www.sinatramd.com

A healthy body is a guest-chamber for the soul; a sick body is a prison. – Francis Bacon
He who has health has hope; and he who has hope, has everything. – Arabian proverb

TIME

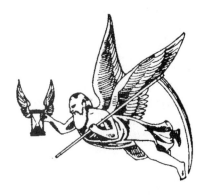

I have just a little minute,
Only sixty seconds in it,
Just a tiny little minute,
Give account if I abuse it;
Forced upon me; can't refuse it
Didn't seek it, didn't choose it,
But it's up to me to use it.
I must suffer if I lose it;
But eternity is in it. – Unknown

67

Senior Foot Steps

As we age, changes in the feet happen naturally. Older feet tend to spread and change shape slightly. You might find your shoes, as a senior, increase by one size to accommodate the gradual spreading. This is normal, as is the reduction in the amount of fatty padding of the soles. The skin often dries and thins on older feet, resulting in cracking and inflammation. This can be reduced or eliminated by using moistening oils and lotions and following this Bragg Foot Culture Program.

With age, blood supply to the feet often diminishes, causing cold feet, fatigue and sometimes numbness. Moderate exercise helps alleviate this common problem.

Arthritis, another common difficulty of ageing, may be felt especially in the feet. Basically, arthritis is a condition affecting various joints. There may be a decrease or increase in space between bones, a break-down of part of a bone, or a growth of bony bumps.

Investing in good, proper fitting shoes will help keep your feet healthy and happy and will add to your overall feeling of well-being. Remember, your feet carry you through life - so be extra loving and caring to them!

20 Year Study Shows Being Fit Saves Money

In 2004 health care costs are soaring up!!! Back in 2003, the average American spent $5,500 on health care. Private health-insurance premiums jumped 8.2% back in 1998, more than doubled as in previous years (3.3% in 1996, 3.5% in 1997). This revealing 20 year study done by Dr. Ted Mitchell of The Cooper Clinic in Texas monitored 6,679 men. Results showed those who exercised more, required fewer doctor visits. Being fit cuts yearly medical expenses 25 to 60%. Study also found all you need to stay fit is to exercise just 20 to 30 minutes a day, four or five days a week. Physically fit people live longer and enjoy a better quality of life! www.cooperaerobics.com

Follow the steps of the Godly instead, and stay on the right path, for good men enjoy life to the full. – Proverbs 2:20-21

Nourish the mind like you would your body. The mind cannot survive on junk food.

As I stride along on my daily three-mile brisk walk, I say to myself – often out loud – "Health, Strength, Youth, Vitality, Understanding, Peace, Joy and Salvation for Eternity." It amazes me daily how our wonderful Lord faithfully fills my life with all His Glorious Blessings! – Patricia Bragg, N.D., Ph.D., Health Crusader

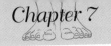

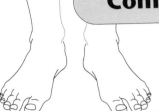

Chapter 7

Common Foot Problems

Arthritis
Effects Over
70 Million Americans

Arthritis is the umbrella term for a complex of diseases which cause the swelling and inflammation of the cartilage and lining of the joints, as well as an increase in joint fluid. The feet are particularly susceptible to arthritis because of the weight they bear and because each foot has so many potentially vulnerable joints.

Over 70 million Americans in a recent U.S. Gov. Survey are afflicted by this painful disease. Arthritis is primarily prevalent in those over 50, but now has victims of all ages, even children. There is some evidence to suggest that it might be hereditary in some manifestations, however, symptoms may appear through viral and bacterial infections – for example the organisms present in gonorrhea, pneumonia and Lyme disease can cause inflammations in the joints. Injuries, especially ignored injuries may lead to arthritic symptoms, and more often in the feet, where injuries most often can go untreated. Although seemingly unrelated, bowel disorders such as colitis and ileitis may also be accompanied by even arthritic symptoms in the ankle and toe joints.

It is important to see a podiatric practitioner if you notice any of th ese symptoms in the feet: swelling, recurring pain, tenderness, redness or heat in a joint; early morning stiffness, limited joint motion and the appearance of rashes and growths on the skin. For latest survey, statistics, etc., visit www.firstgov.gov

Your arteries are living structures with vital functions! Their linings have about 98 different enzymatic systems, whose purpose is not only to prevent blockage damage, but to allow oxygen and nutrients to permeate freely through them into the heart muscle and other tissues. – Dr. Savely Yurkovsky, Cardiologist

Rheumatoid Arthritis

Rheumatoid arthritis is the most crippling and serious form of the disease. It is a complex, systematic disorder which affects multiple joints over the entire body. 90% of Rheumatoid arthritis sufferers experience symptoms in the feet and ankles, the most common of which are pain, stiffness and swelling. The toes twist and stiffen into positions called hammer toe or claw toe. As RA affects the various systems in the body, one may simultaneously experience fatigue, fever, loss of appetite and weight loss. Women are 3 to 4 times more likely to suffer from Rheumatoid arthritis than men.

Osteo Arthritis

There are more than 100 varieties of arthritis of which Osteoarthritis, or degenerative joint disease, is the most common form. Osteoarthritis usually develops gradually with age, as wear and tear on bones sees the cartilage covering become worn and frayed. The symptoms include swelling, pain and inflammation. Occasionally joint injuries can cause the sudden onset of pain. Osteoarthritis can also develop months or years after an injury. Being overweight exacerbates arthritic symptoms as the excess weight accelerates deterioration of cartilage.

Gout

Gout is a form of arthritis and millions (mostly are men), suffer from this painful condition. Gout is brought on by a buildup of uric acid mainly in the foot joints, usually affects a single big toe joint but also can affect joints throughout the body. Normally associated with diets rich in red meat, organ meats (brains, kidney, liver, etc.) heavy sauces, coffee and alcohol. Foods to avoid are heavy oily foods such as anchovies, mackerel, sardines, mussels and nuts roasted in oil. Enjoy foods like starchy organic vegetables, corn, fruits, soy products, tofu, etc. Stop all white sugar and refined flour products. A paste made of cayenne oil & wintergreen oil applied to sore areas helps relieve pain and inflammation. There is also a hereditary element to the disease.

Arthritis and Gout Foot Treatments

Conservative foot treatments for arthritis and also gout, includes healthy diet, fasting, weight control and proper shoes. Try keeping the area mobile and more flexible. Exercising, especially in a pool is particularly beneficial. In water you weigh less, put less strain on the joints and you are more flexible. It's also very important to maintain good body posture and foot balance to reduce stress on the joints.

GOUT PAIN

Herbal teas such as Yarro, Willow Bark, Dandelion and Burdock are known to help relieve arthritis and gout pains. Taking Vitamin C, CoQ10 and MSM is helpful. Garlic (fresh is best) boosts the immune system and helps reduce pain. Reduce the fat in your diet and cut out meat, salt, sugar, coffee, alcohol and junk fast foods!

For a list of homeopathic pain relievers for gout and arthritic pain and stiffness relievers see website: *www.holisticonline.com/Remedies/Arthritis/arth_homeopathy.htm*

As a last resort there are various surgical procedures available. **Arthroscopic Debridement** can be beneficial in the earlier stages of arthritic development. The arthroscope, a tiny instrument with a lens, camera and lighting system is inserted into the problem joint. The image is relayed onto a monitor and the surgeon can get an idea of what needs to be done. The joint can be cleaned, and growths and any excess bone can gently be removed with tiny knives, forceps and shavers.

Arthrodesis is done only in the most drastic cases! This surgery procedure does away with the joint altogether, and fuses the bones permanently. The bones are held together with screws, plates and pins until the healing is complete.

Joint replacement, or **Arthroplasty** may be carried out in only rare cases! Artificial implants are used to replace ankle joints. This procedure however, isn't as successful as hip or knee replacements, and additional surgery may be required.

Ankle and foot surgery of any kind can be painful and involve long recuperation periods. One should keep the foot elevated above the level of the heart for the first few days. You will not be able to put full weight on your foot for several weeks and full healing recovery may take months. Physical therapy exercises and gentle massage are an important part of the recovery process. Within 3 to 4 months the patient may return to normal activities, sometimes with aid of special shoes, orthotics or braces.

For more Foot Care info on web see:
- *orthoinfo.aaos.org*
- *www.apma.org/topics/Arthritis.htm*
- *www.webterrace.com/home/ad.htm*
- *www.celebrex.com/4_1_daily_living.asp*

Achilles Tendonitis

The Achilles tendon is the largest tendon in the body, and the most frequently ruptured tendon by athletes and sports people (page 101). Achilles Tendonitis is a condition triggered by suddenly increasing running speed, by rapid running after a period of non-sporting activity and by not warming up and stretching before running. Another common cause of Achilles Tendonitis is over-pronation (like flat feet) when the foot arch collapses upon bearing too much weight, resulting in added stress being placed on the Achilles Tendon.

Symptoms include pain in morning during first steps of the day. Pain after exercise usually begins mildly and often becomes progressively worse, with sluggishness in foot and leg movement.

Best Treatment is rest, ample water, supplements, MSM, etc. Stop sport and all activity for at least 2–4 weeks, and try swimming as a non-aggravating alternative to regular exercise habits. If not improving, wear foot boot to help restrict foot activity so it can heal.

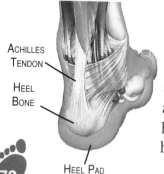

ACHILLES TENDON

HEEL BONE

HEEL PAD

You cannot put the same shoe on every foot.
– Pubilius Syrus

All is born of water, all is sustained by pure water. – Goethe

Shoe Orthotics and inner shoe cushions: These help damaged areas and provide some relief from discomfort (page 95). After rest period, stretching should be introduced to maintain flexibility and promote strength. Surgery as always, should be a last resort and only after wise advise.

Preventative Steps: Always walk, stretch and warm up before running, making increases in running speed gradually – in increments of no more than 10% per week, always choosing running footwear carefully and replacing regularly (see pages 93-96). For more ideas and info see web: *www.foot.com/html/achilles_tend.html* or *orthoinfo.aaos.org*

NORMAL FOOT 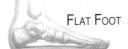 FLAT FOOT

Flat feet, or over-pronation, is what happens when the arches of the feet collapse due to a number of factors, including weight bearing, obesity, pregnancy and repeated contact of the plantar, or base of the foot, with hard surfaces. It can also be a hereditary condition. As the framework of the foot caves in, extra stress is placed on other parts of the foot. Heel Spurs, Plantar Fasciitis and Tendonitis, among other ailments, may result. In many cases of over-pronation, initially no discomfort may be experienced, however, over time there will be an onset of pain, which in turn can even make walking uncomfortable! Problems can be relayed to the calves, shins and knees. **The best treatment for flat feet is the use of correct orthotics that you can insert in your shoes,** *www.goodfeet.com*. They should be supportive and feel comfortable in arch area. Always choose footwear with care to ensure comfortable fit (see pages 90-92). For more ideas check this website: *www.foot.com*

Diabetes and Foot Problems

Diabetes Mellitus is a disease which brings about the inability of the body to produce insulin, or convert sugars, starches and other foods into energy. High blood sugar levels are a result, the long term effects of which are damage to the feet, kidneys, blood vessels, eyes, heart and nerves. Symptoms include slow to heal wounds, blurred vision, fatigue, excessive weight loss, hunger and thirst, frequent urination and even numbness of hands

73

and feet. The causes of diabetes is unknown, but we strongly feel it's lifestyle, diet and habits and processed, hi-sugar foods and beverages, etc. that most often trigger the problems! Most doctors say there is no known cure, but famous Dr. Dean Ornish, advisor to presidents, etc. (*www.ornish.com*) says with dietary changes and exercise, diabetics can improve and may keep the serious symptoms at bay. Self-testing for blood sugar levels is an important measure in warding off complications.(www.diabetes.com)

There are two types of diabetes: Type 1 which occurs most frequently in children and adolescents and is caused by the inability of the pancreas to produce the necessary insulin, and Type 2 or adult onset diabetes, which affects 90-95% of cases, who inject insulin or take oral medication to control the disease.

Diabetes Nerve Disease is a complication which affects 60-70% of people with diabetes. Foot ulcers and gangrene effect about 15% of diabetics, of which between 15 and 25% require amputation and there is a 50% likelihood of a further amputation, within 5 years. There are over 86,000 such operations performed on diabetics yearly, also a high 39-60% mortality rate within 5 years. (*Dr. Linus Pauling saved limbs with daily 2-3 hour slow IV drip of 30 to 50 gram Vit. "C" and also Chelation Treatments work miracles. See web: www.acam.org for Chelation doctors in your area.*)

Foot Ulceration

Ulceration may also be caused by poorly fitting shoes or something as simple as a rubbing stocking seam. As skin sensation is diminished, a wound can quickly develop unnoticed. A foot podiatric physician can help prevent and treat such wounds. There are remarkable new scientific developments - new substances, which have the feel and texture of human skin which may be applied to the problem area. There are also many preventative measures the diabetic can take to diminish the risk of ulcers and other complications in this book.

A Yale University Study showed that raw honey helped cure skin ulcers and bedsores better than any other medication.

The treatment of diseases should go to the root cause, and most often it is found in severe body dehydration from lack of sufficient pure distilled or purified water. Also, in living an unhealthy lifestyle!

Prevent Diabetic Foot Problems

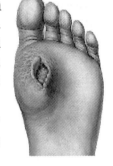

① Wash feet morning and night with mild soap and lukewarm water (never hot). Diabetics should not do foot soaks as skin can become soft and more vulnerable. With a soft towel dry carefully, using cornstarch or tea tree powder to keep feet dry.

② Check your feet and toes daily for sores, cuts and bruises. Inspect the toenails for changes in coloration or thickening.

③ Keep your body as healthy and fit as possible and your weight normal to reduce any likelihood of future diabetic complications! Many diabetics tend to overeat and become overweight! *www.aofas.org/carediabetic.asp*

④ If a smoker, stop now to reduce risks of circulatory problems, and don't drink alcohol! Drinking accelerates the development of diabetic problems and causes numb feet, creating a possible serious risk of undetected injury.

⑤ Exercise is an excellent way to improve circulation and keep weight down. Walking is the best exercise for diabetics. Wearing comfortable sport shoes are important.

⑥ Wear thick, soft socks and choose well fitted shoes (see pages 90-92). High heels, boots and all shoes with pointed toes should be avoided! Don't wear tight, constricting leg wear. Don't walk barefoot especially outdoors, to avoid cuts and any possible infection!

⑦ Don't try to remove calluses or corns yourself as many preparations can burn and even scar the skin.

⑧ Trim toenails straight across, avoid cutting corners. Use an emery board to gently smooth any rough corners.

⑨ Have regular foot checkups with your foot doctor. For more interesting info on web: *Diabetes.com or orthoinfo.org*

What are Amino Acids? They're the building blocks of all our organs and tissues. They are the building blocks of proteins. They are essential for the production of energy within ourselves, for detoxification and for the vital transmission of nerve impulses. In short, they are the very soup of life, and they are almost always overlooked and neglected. – Henry J. Hoegerman, M.D. A Health Pioneer who favors using Bragg Liquid Aminos, wrote this about our delicious all-purpose seasoning from certified Non-GMO healthy soybeans.

Bunions

A bunion is a large, sore bump on the joint which connects the big toe to the foot (metatarsophalangeal or MTP joint). The toe is forced to bend towards the other toes causing an enlargement of the bone. This is a painful condition, and as the joint carries much of the bodies weight, the pain can become chronic if left untreated. The second toe may be pushed out of alignment and also arthritis may develop. Bunions, which are caused predominantly by the wearing of tight, constricting shoes, boots and high heels, are more common in women than in men. More than 50% of older women in the United States have bunions and foot problems.

A smaller painful lump on the outside of the foot at the base of the little toe is called a **bunionette**. It should be treated, in the same way as a big toe bunion.

Although foot problems and faulty foot mechanics can be hereditary, it is bad habits such as the wearing of narrow, ill-fitting pointed shoes that is the cause of most bunions in 90% of cases. Other causes are congenital deformities, neuromuscular disorders and foot injuries. Most ballet dancers are prone to developing bunions for example. Arthritis sufferers, people with flat feet or low heel arches and even cowboy boot wearers are also at serious risk.

Prevention is always better than the treatment!

Choose comfortable shoes that conform to the size of your foot, preferably with a wide instep and broad toe box (see pages 90-92). **Never force your foot into a shoe that is too small, too short and too tight!!!** Avoid all sharply pointed shoes and heels of more than 2 inches.

If you already have a bunion, for relief you can apply a non-medicated bunion pad around the bony protrudence. Shoe inserts may be helpful for reducing pain and for preventing symptoms from worsening. See more info page 95. If the bunion becomes inflamed, apply ice packs several times daily to reduce swelling and pain. It's wise to seek professional podiatric advice if pain continues.

It's a little known fact that about 80% of sodium we eat comes not from salt we add at the table or during cooking, but from processed, packaged foods.
– Tufts University Nutrition Letter, www.healthletter.tufts.edu

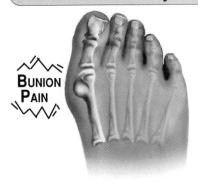

BUNION
PAIN

Should **bunion** surgery be required, several procedures are offered. In a simple bunion-ectomy the surgeon removes just the bony protruberance. More severe cases might require a more complex procedure involving the cutting of the bone and joint realignment. Bunion surgery is generally done on the same day, outpatient basis. However, recovery can be a slow process! **Caution:** Get at least three opinions from board certified orthopedic doctors! For more foot info see web: *orthoinfo.aaos.org* or *www.apma.org/topics/bunions.htm*

Hammertoes

Hammertoes are the bending of one of the 2nd to 5th toes at the middle joint - the proximal inter-phalangeal joint - a deformity caused by improperly fitting shoes or a muscle imbalance in foot and toes. The abnormal balance causes pressure on the joints and tendons, finally resulting in a contraction. The toe takes on a V, or hammer shape. The condition may also be hereditary, brought on by trauma, or even arthritis.

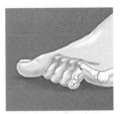

Flexible Hammertoes the condition in early stages, because they are still moveable at the joint and more easily treatable with hammertoe splints, proper shoes, orthotics, etc. If allowed to develop into **Rigid Hammertoes** the situation becomes more serious. Joints become misaligned and immobile, the tendons tight, and often the only remaining recourse is toe surgery.

The first, most effective conservative treatment should be to wear shoes with soft, deep and roomy toe boxes (pages 90-92). Wearing high heels should absolutely be avoided. A non-medicated hammertoe pad (drscholls.com) may be applied around the bony prominence to decrease pressure on area. If the hammertoe becomes inflamed, ice packs may be applied several times daily. A podiatric physician may also be able to suggest certain exercises to stretch and strengthen muscles such as picking objects up (pencils, marbles) off the floor with your toes.

Should all conservative measures fail, hammertoes can be corrected by surgery (again, get 3 opinions) which is usually carried out, using local anesthetic, on an outpatient basis. For more hammertoe information on the web visit: *www.apma.org/topics/hammertoes.htm* or *orthoinfo.aaos.org*

Foot Corns

Corns are a build up of dead skin cells, usually located on the top or inside of the toe, which form hardened areas containing a central cone shape core which may push down on the nerves underneath generating pain (see page 64). A very common ailment, corns are formed by friction against a tight fitting shoe for example. The bones of the toe press against the shoe creating pressure on the skin. If left unchecked corns can become inflamed and extremely sore.

Sometimes corns appear between the toes, known as soft corns, they are the result of bony protruberances rubbing against each other and corns stay soft due to perspiration.

Prevention of foot corns is relatively simple. Always wear well fitted shoes with deep and wide toe boxes. Buy shoes made from materials which breathe and are flexible such as leather, canvas, etc. (see pages 90-92), wear cotton socks and wash feet often, drying well afterwards.

To treat already existent corns, soak feet in a bowl of vinegar water regularly to soften corn and use a pumice stone to lightly brush away dead skin cells. Wear a corn pad over the problem area to relieve pressure. Placing a piece of lambs wool between the toes helps cushion soft corns. Applying petroleum jelly or lanolin-enriched hand lotion helps keep skin soft, but corn removing ointments that contain acid can damage healthy skin. They should never be used by pregnant women or by people who are diabetic or who have poor circulation.

Your foot doctor will be able to help control corns by carefully trimming them, however this should not be carried out at home, especially by diabetics! For more foot care information see these important websites: *www.foot.com/info/cond_corns.jsp* or *orthoinfo.aaos.org*

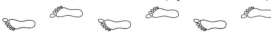

Foot Calluses

Calluses are similar formations of thick, hard, dead skin which are usually found on the ball-of-the-foot, the heel and outside of the big toe (see also page 63). Some have centers known as nucleations which can be painful when pressed. Similarly to corns, calluses are formed due to continual friction or pressure from tight fitting or high heeled and pointed shoes, being overweight, having flat feet or due to lack of sufficient fat padding or caused by an abusive walking gait and posture.

Calluses are natures way of protecting the area beneath the skin. Calluses also appear on the hands for example, but in a useful protective capacity. Musicians who play stringed instruments find it a painful occupation until thick calluses appear on the fingertips to protect them. In countries where people go barefoot for much of the time, a thick and useful layer of callus forms on the feet to offer similar protection! However in western society where the wearing of shoes is normal, calluses are usually symptoms of mechanical problems, and will continue to aggravate and cause discomfort until the problem is corrected!

Proper orthotics are an effective way of giving relief to pressure points by redistributing weight equally around the foot. Soak the feet in warm vinegar water, dry well and gently rub away the dead skin with a pumice stone. Again, no cutting or trimming with knives or razor blades should be carried out by anyone (especially diabetics) but only done by a qualified podiatrist! For more website info about calluses,etc see: *www.foot.com/info/cond_ calluses.jsp* or *www.podiatrychannel.com/calluses/selfhelp.shtml*

Athlete's Foot

Athlete's Foot is a skin condition, usually occurring between the toes, caused by a fungus which thrives in warm, moist conditions (see also page 18). The fungus proliferates on the feet because shoes create the ideal dark and humid environment. Swimming pools, showers and locker rooms are also breeding grounds for the fungi, and it is in such places that it is transferred from one person to another.

Athlete's Foot Plagues Millions

Athlete's foot is so named because the fungal infection is most common among athletes. Millions suffer from it who frequent gyms, swimming pools, etc. Symptoms include itchy, scaly, inflamed, cracked skin and blisters. When blisters break and the raw underskin is exposed then the pain and discomfort increases. If the infection is scratched, it can spread to other parts of the foot, the soles and toenails, as well as to other body parts such as the underarms and groin. Athlete's foot can also be spread to other areas of the body by contaminated towels, clothing and bed sheets.

To avoid contracting the disease, avoid walking barefoot in communal showers (wear rubber sandals). To control symptoms, wear light shoes or thongs, change socks frequently and use cornstarch to reduce any perspiration.

Tips to Help Banish Athlete's Foot:

• Soak feet daily in Bragg Organic Vinegar (2 Tbsps) warm water in shallow pan to help banish athlete's foot and fungus. Repeat daily until rash subsides.
• Soak feet in warm water with 2 Tbsps each of salt and Bragg Organic Vinegar in shallow pan.
• Apply baking soda paste to fungus between toes for 1 to 2 hours, wear white cotton socks after applying. Prepare paste with few drops of Bragg Vinegar to Tbsp of baking soda. After treatment: Rinse, dry and dust area with cornstarch (*optional add ⅓ tsp garlic powder*). For web info: *www.apma.org/topics/athfoot.htm*

Foot Odors

There are two principal reasons for malodorous feet, feet sweat and are usually encased in shoes (see page 98). Bacteria thrives in socks and shoes where a combination of darkness and temperatures which can reach 102°F, that creates the perfect breeding ground. The greater amount of moisture, the more bacteria is generated. In turn bacteria produces a substance called Isovaleric Acid which is the source of most foot odors condition called hyperhidrosis that can generally affects males. Wear well-ventalated shoes, sandals or sneekers with breathing holes to allow feet to breathe and be healthy.

He who wears the shoe, best knows where it pinches. – Norwegian saying

It is important to practice good foot hygiene to keep bacteria levels down. Soak your feet daily in warm soapy water for approximately 10 minutes. Dry thoroughly afterwards. Apply cornstarch powder. Change shoes and socks everyday. Alternate shoes, don't wear the same pair two days in a row. Wear shoes made from materials that allow feet to breathe such as leather or canvas. It's best to avoid nylon socks and plastic shoes.

Soak feet in strong black tea for 30 minutes per day for a week. The tannic acid in the black tea will help kill the bacteria. Use four tea bags per pint of water, boil mixture for 15 minutes, then add two quarts of cool water. Soak feet in warm brew. For more foot care info, check out website: *orthoinfo.aaos.org*

Heel Pain and Fractures

Heel pain is one of the most common problems that affects the foot. It's usually caused by walking gait abnormalities which place too much stress on the heel bone, or by heavy pounding of the feet on hard surfaces such as concrete, either while playing sports, or simply by wearing shoes which offer little or not sufficient cushioning (see pages 90-92). Pain is nature's warning signal, telling us that if we don't pay attention to it, problems will follow! Usually heel pain will go away on its own accord if one refrains from the activities or shoes which caused the pain and when the foot is given rest.

Inflamed Achilles Tendon

If you have pain behind the heel, the area where the Achilles Tendon inserts into the heel bone, it may be inflamed (see page 72). The heel bone is the largest of the 26 bones in the feet. This can be caused by too much running or from wearing shoes which dig into the heel. Stop sporting activity for a period and resting the foot would be beneficial. Stretching exercises may also help – with the foot flat on the floor, lean forward against a wall until a stretch can be felt.

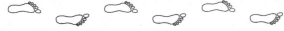

Medicine is only palliative, for behind disease lies the cause and this cause no drug can reach. – Dr. Weir Mitchell

Plantar Fasciitis

If you experience pain beneath the heel you may have an inflamed fascia - the tissue band which connects the heel bone to the base of the toes, 'plantar' meaning bottom of the foot. Again, this can be caused by a lot of running or jumping. Rest, gentle exercise and stretching are the first recourse, and the wearing of a cushioned heel pads in the shoes may also be beneficial.

Heel Spurs

Another major cause of heel pain is the heel spur – a bony growth (calcium deposit) which can extend up to half an inch on the inside of the heel (see also page 66). It is flat and wide in shape, rather like a shelf and is only visible using an x-ray. Heel spurs occur when plantar fascia is strained over a long period of time, especially when Plantar Fasciitis goes ignored. Sporting activity is another major cause, as are shoes which offer inappropriate support (see pages 90-92), weight changes and obesity. The condition will generally improve greatly with rest, the application of ice and periodic stretching. However, rest is a course of action which should be undertaken for short periods only, as muscular atrophy may result and may in turn only contribute to the problem. **As always, surgery should be a last resort**. For further information on Heel Spurs and Plantar Fasciitis see excellent and extensive website: *heelspurs.com*

Heel Fractures

It is very difficult to break the heel bone due to its thickness and positioning in the foot. If such an injury has been sustained, the foot should be elevated and dressed to prevent bones shifting. Ice packs should be applied every hour or so for 20 minutes to reduce any swelling. The healing period could be in the region of six to eight weeks, and possibly longer in some cases.

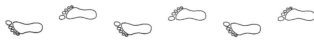

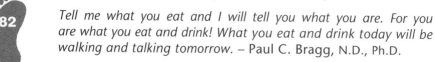

Tell me what you eat and I will tell you what you are. For you are what you eat and drink! What you eat and drink today will be walking and talking tomorrow. – Paul C. Bragg, N.D., Ph.D.

If the bones have not been dislodged by the force of the injury, surgery may not be necessary. However, if they have been shifted out of place you might need surgery. You will not be able to put any weight on the heel for usually 8 -10 weeks after surgery. For more information do visit web: *orthoinfo.aaos.org or www.apma.org/topics/heel.htm*

Morton's Neuroma

A neuroma is a benign growth, or thickening of nerve tissue surrounding the digital nerve between the third and fourth toes. It is caused by an abnormal function of the foot causing the bones to squeeze the nerve at this point. Symptoms include pain, burning and even numbness in the area. It is commonly described as the awkward feeling of 'walking on a marble'.

The main factors that contribute to the formation of a neuroma are deformities such as flat feet or high arches, which place abnormal stress on the toe joints. The wearing of high heels, boots and constricting footwear that causes the toes to be squeezed together, this is what promotes injury and stress to the foot.

The first step in treatment or prevention is to wear roomy and comfortable footwear that allow the bones to spread out and please avoid high heels (pages 90-92). Custom shoe orthotics may help many to relieve pain by supporting and separating the bones. Foot soaks and massage are effective in temporary pain relief, as is rest. Ice pack (*20 minutes on and off*) may be applied to dull pain.

For more severe and long term cases, surgery may be necessary. The procedure to remove the enlarged nerve is usually carried out on an outpatient basis. The recovery time may be several weeks. For more info on web see: *www.foot.com/html/morton_neur.html or www.apma.org/topics/neuromas.htm or orthoinfo.aaos.org*

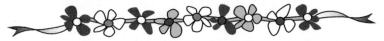

Fasting is an effective and safe method of detoxifying the body – a technique used for centuries for healing. Fast regularly one day a week and help the body cleanse and heal itself to stay well. When a cold or illness is coming on, or even depression – it's best to fast! Bragg Books were my conversion to the healthy way.
– James Balch, M.D. Co-Author of Prescription for Nutritional Healing

Ingrown Toenails

This extremely common ailment is often caused by trimming your toenails too short and rounding off the corner to match the shape of the toe while doing so. What happens is that this 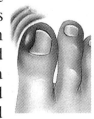 encourages the toenail to grow into the skin of the toe, often curling as it does so and embedding downwards (page 65). The area around the nail will become sore and tender, later possibly becoming infected and very painful. If left unattended the skin may begin to grow over the nail. Usually the big toe is affected. Wearing shoes that are too tight is another cause, and heredity also can play a part.

To prevent ingrown toenails always trim nails straight across, not longer than the tips of the toes, using toenail clippers. Don't wear shoes which are too tight and that press on the toenails (see Chapter 8) and keep feet clean.

Treatment for an ingrowing toenail should begin with soaking foot in warm vinegar water several times per day. Cleanliness is of upmost importance. Gently lift edge of toenail and insert cotton underneath – change dressing regularly. Wear sandals if possible. If the problem recurs, or if you are in pain see your podiatrist who may be able to remove part of the problem nail.

Fungal Nails

Onychomycosis, or fungal infection of the nail may be present for years without causing discomfort, and for this reason often goes ignored (see also page 99). The toenails can often gradually change color and texture, becoming thick, dark and foul smelling. This infection is caused by fungal organisms underneath the surface of the nail. This may spread to other toenails, the skin and even the fingernails.

The fungi thrive in damp environments such as showers, swimming pools and locker rooms – places where people are likely to be walking barefoot.

Those who suffer from chronic conditions such as circulatory problems and diabetes are particularly susceptible to these fungal problems. To prevent fungal nails, as with ingrown toenails, toenails should be cut straight across using nail clippers. Cleanliness is the best prevention against infection. Wash the feet with soapy vinegar water on a regular basis, drying thoroughly. Change socks and shoes more than once per day. Wear well fitting shoes made of a material which breathes, such as leather and canvas (see pages 90-92), and wear shower shoes when using public showers.

A mild infection may be temporarily suppressed by a daily vinegar cleansing routine, however symptoms may return. It is always best to catch any such infection in its early stages, so visit your pediatrician who will advise the best course of action to take. In some extreme cases surgery may be required. For more information on the web see: *www.apma.org/topics/nail.htm or orthoinfo.aaos.org*

Chiropractic Solutions for Foot Problems

The feet are extremely susceptible to disorders for many reasons. They are complex machines, containing some 26 bones, 33 movable joints and a host of ligaments, nerves and blood vessels. They bear the constant weight of our bodies and have to withstand the constant abuse dealt to them through walking and running.

Perhaps the most common type of injury is the ankle sprain, but the range of problems threatening the feet is wide, running from a simple stubbed toe or blister to a torn ligament or fracture. Foot pain can arise from badly fitting footwear, from bad walking habits such as favoring one foot over the other, from unevenly distributing bodyweight as well as from sports injuries.

In the same way that foot problems may originate in other body parts, disorders may cause a chain reaction of dysfunctions throughout the body. When you modify your gait and posture due to foot misalignment or malfunction your body may be forced to try and overcompensate, leading to a variety of knee, hip, back and even shoulder problems, even to painful headaches.

What is Chiropractic?

If you suffer from foot disorders and pain it would be a good idea to consult a chiropractor, who will be experienced in the relief of pain, and the correction of skeletal and connecting tissue misalignments. Everyone is at risk of suffering foot trouble, however, particularly susceptible are diabetics, athletes, dancers, overweight and older citizens.

Chiropractic, which is derived from the Greek words 'chiros' and 'praktikos' which mean 'done by hand', looks at the relationship between the spinal column, the skeletal system and the connecting soft tissue and nerves in the restoration and maintenance of health. It was developed by a Canadian, Dr. Daniel David Palmer in Davenport, Iowa who performed the first chiropractic adjustment on September 18, 1885. However, cruder forms of physical manipulation had been practiced for thousands of years in ancient Greece, Rome, India and the Orient. Even Hippocrates, the father of modern medicine used such methods of healing way back in 400 B.C.

It's very common during a lifetime, that one will experience a strain or sprain of the foot or ankle. Over time the soft tissues may heal, however the bones may remain misaligned. Discomfort and complications may continue and could be contributed to a misalignment. Often after one body trauma has been experienced, others follow. This is probably for the same reason.

Treating pain with pain killers is not the right solution, finding out the root cause of the problem is wiser and more effective! This is where chiropractic comes in to examine and if needed, take an x-ray and then the treatment will be decided upon. Chiropractic foot adjustments can bring pain relief and restore function. They can prevent problems from spreading from the feet to knees, hips, lower and upper back, the neck and other areas of the body. For a selection of case histories of chiropractic treatment for a wide range of leg, hip and foot ailments see this website: *www.chiroweb.com/find/hips.html.*

Natural Healthy Foods Prevent Osteoporosis

When we were doing nutritional research along the Adriatic coast of Italy, we found *ageless* men and women, advanced in calendar years but whose bodies were youthful, supple and their bones firm, strong and resilient. Their diet consisted primarily of organically grown fresh salads, properly cooked vegetables, olive oil, dark breads, pasta and natural cheeses rich in calcium, minerals, and vitamins, all essential for strong bones. In our extensive research on nutrition, we never found osteoporosis among active people who lived on a simple diet of *live*, natural healthy foods (see web: *www.calciuminfo.com*).

The American fast, trash diet, in addition to lacking vitamins and minerals, is highly acid-producing, due to high proportion of refined white sugar, flour and animal proteins, which increase body acidity with an adverse effect on bones. Strong bones require alkaline balance in the body which is naturally maintained with a healthy diet of raw organic fruits and vegetables.

The worst villain is refined white sugar and its many products; there is no single food more devastating to the spine and other bones of the entire body. It leaches calcium, phosphorus, magnesium and manganese out of the bones, making them weak, porous and brittle. Candy, sweets and refined white sugar products and drinks are also prime causes of tooth decay. Since teeth are the body's hardest tissue, you can understand what refined white sugar does to other bones and cartilages (protective cushions between bones) of the skeletal system, including your spinal column (see web: *www.homocysteine.com*).

To maintain good health, normal weight and increase the good life of radiant health, joy and happiness, the body must be exercised properly (stretching, walking, jogging, running, biking, swimming, deep breathing, good posture, etc.) and nourished wisely with healthy foods. – Paul C. Bragg

---

Do most humans get all their nutritional needs the body requires to operate at top performance? Virtually no one's diet provides them with 100% of all the nutrients needed. To ensure and help replenish the essential vitamins, minerals and trace minerals the body needs, it is wise to take daily supplements. – JAMA, Reports

Locations in the Body Where Osteoporosis, Arthritis, Pain and Misery Hit the Hardest

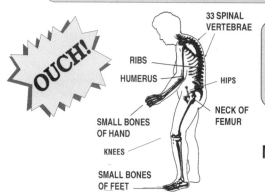

33 SPINAL VERTEBRAE
RIBS
HUMERUS
HIPS
NECK OF FEMUR
SMALL BONES OF HAND
KNEES
SMALL BONES OF FEET

OUCH!

OSTEOPOROSIS
Affects over 30 Million and Kills 400,000 Americans Annually

Boron
Miracle Trace Mineral For Healthy Bones

BORON – A trace mineral for healthier bones that also helps the body absorb more vital calcium, minerals and necessary hormones! Good sources are most vegetables, fresh and sun- dried fruits, prunes, raw nuts, soybeans and nutritional Brewer's yeast. The U.S. Department of Agriculture's Human Nutrition Lab in Grand Forks, North Dakota, says boron is usually found in soil and in foods, but many Americans eat a diet low in boron. They conducted a 17 week study which showed a daily 3 to 6 mgs boron supplement enabled participants to reduce loss (demineralization) of calcium, phosphorus and magnesium from their bodies. This loss is usually caused by eating refined, processed fast foods and lots of meat, salt, sugar and fat and a dietary lack of fresh vegetables, fruits and whole grains *(www.all-natural.com)*.

After 8 weeks on boron, participants' calcium loss was cut 40%. It also helped double important hormone levels vital in maintaining calcium and healthy bones. Millions of women on estrogen therapy for osteoporosis* may want to use boron, a healthier choice. Also consider natural progesterone (2%) raw yam cream and other natural options. For pain, joint support and healing use a glucosamine/chondriotin/MSM combo *(caps, liquid and roll-on)*.

University of Wales recent study showed Cod Liver Oil eases pain and heals. Scientific studies also show women benefit from a healthy lifestyle that includes some gentle sunshine and ample exercise *(even weightlifting)* to maintain healthier bones, combined with a low-fat, high-fiber, natural carbohydrates and fresh salads, greens, vegetable, fruit diet and also add 2 tsp cinnamon powder to teas, drinks, etc. This lifestyle helps protect against heart disease, high blood pressure, cancer and many other ailments. I'm happy to see science now agrees with my Dad who first stated these health truths over 80 years ago!

* *For more hormone and osteoporosis facts read pioneer Dr. John Lee's book. What Your Doctor May Not Tell You About Menopause. www.amazon.com*

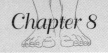

Chapter 8

Your Shoes Are Important

When You Cannot Go Barefoot...

Although going barefoot is best for your feet, it is not always possible, or safe, to walk around certain areas without shoes. Sometimes even exercising your feet in the most natural way, walking barefoot on a beautiful sandy beach or grassy (*hopefully toxic free*) lawns of a park, at times can be dangerous. Unfortunately, many most popular beaches are often marred by broken bottles, rusted tin cans, etc., so know the area where you are walking and remember caution (watch where you step) is essential.

It is extremely important to treat your feet to the best shoes available! There are many fine shoes on the market that have been scientifically designed to provide the most natural support for busy, active feet, no matter what they are doing; sitting, walking, standing, jogging, biking, aerobics or competing in a marathon or triathlon!

Check the Yellow Pages of the phone book under *Shoes* for a specialty sports shoe store. These shops sell shoes that are geared for any activity you might wish to undertake, including hiking, tennis and a variety of other sports. Shoes for each of these sports are developed to compensate for any possible stress on different foot parts.

For example, the walking shoe is specially cushioned at the heel to protect the foot and the leg from impact at the point of contact with the ground to avoid excess jarring. Hiking shoes or boots are usually steel reinforced around the toe box and ankle to prevent rubbing, stubbing and the possibility of injury from sharp rocks and sticks which are often encountered on hiking trails.

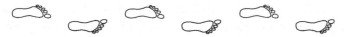

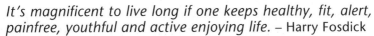

It's magnificent to live long if one keeps healthy, fit, alert, painfree, youthful and active enjoying life. – Harry Fosdick

Getting the Proper Shoe Fit

Investing in good, proper fitting shoes will help keep your feet healthy and happy and will add to your overall feeling of well-being. Remember, your feet carry you through life - so be extra loving and caring to them!

Getting the proper fit is not a hit-or-miss situation. There are basic guidelines you can follow when buying shoes. But the most important rule is this: **If the shoe doesn't feel comfortable,** that is, provide the support and cushioning you need, **please keep looking!**

Don't waste your money and threaten your well-being just because you're in a hurry or because the shoe looks pretty. Plan ahead. Buy shoes well before you need them for a special event, whether it be a party, a big hike or a triathlon. A race could be lost with the wrong new shoes - we have seen it happen when we trained athletes! You may need time to break the shoes in. Haste often makes waste when buying shoes. Plan your shoe needs ahead of time and shop wisely! Your feet carry you thru life!

The best possible shoe you can buy is one that is lightweight with a flat heel simulating the bare foot. It should be made of a natural material that is flexible. The best shoe materials are leather (including suede) or canvas. Leather adapts or molds itself to the shape of your foot and generally lasts a longer time than other materials. Canvas, such as that used in many sports shoes, has the same flexibility. Both materials absorb moisture that helps reduce fungus infections and the discomfort and embarrassment of foot perspiration.

Avoid shoes that are made of plastic or other man-made materials. Such shoes most often will not provide the proper foot support. Also your feet can't breathe in plastic!

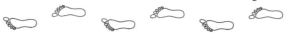

Wear proper fitting footwear at all times as there are over 280 different foot ailments that can be suffered. – American Podiatric Medical Association

---

The world is moving so fast now-a-days that the man who says it can't be done is generally interrupted by someone doing it. – Elbert Hubbard

---

90

True wisdom consists in not departing from Mother Nature, but molding our conduct according to her wise laws. – Seneca

Socks of Natural Materials are Best!

Not only shoes, but socks also, should be made of natural materials, either cotton or wool or a blend of the two. Silk, another natural material from which socks are made, can be worn under other socks in extremely cold weather. Socks made of synthetic fabrics don't absorb perspiration and this keeps the feet trapped in moisture. A warm, wet environment is conducive to the growth of bacteria and fungi and is especially to be avoided during strenuous exercise when the feet perspire profusely. Wearing socks made of synthetics, especially when they are worn all day, can result in fungus infections and in cracking and bleeding between toes.

Custom Molded Shoes

Custom molded shoes are made from an exact plaster cast of your foot. These are particularly beneficial for people who suffer with high insteps, fallen arches or foot genetic problems. Although they are expensive, molded shoes are well constructed with flexible soles and should provide good service for several years with normal use. In most cases, the manufacturer will provide a guarantee that the shoe will survive the usual wear and tear for a certain period of time. Be sure to check on guarantees if you are in the market for a molded shoe. Also, be sure to seek out a reputable manufacturer who takes careful measurements of your feet and makes a working plaster cast. Some better shoes, short of molded shoes and special orthopedic shoes, are the Birkenstock and Ecco brands, which follow the natural foot curve- but be sure the sole is flexible! They come in a wide variety of sandal and shoe styles and most styles will pamper your feet in the most natural way, short of going barefoot. Also, lately in some models, the soles are too stiff which hinders the foot's flexibility.

Life is learning which rules to obey, which rules not to obey, and the wisdom to tell the difference between the two.

There are only two ways to live your life. One is as though nothing is a miracle. The other is as though everything is a miracle. – Albert Einstein

91

How to Buy Comfortable, Healthy Shoes

Wisely buy shoes after carefully trying on the shoes that first seem to meet your various uses and needs (sports, casual, work, dress, etc.). Shopping for shoes in the late afternoon or early evening will help you get an accurate fit, as your feet tend to be slightly larger after spending the day on them. Also, with age and usually during pregnancy, feet tend to get larger. Remember, most people have one foot larger than the other, make sure the salesperson measures both feet and fits the shoes to the larger one. Remember, how your feet feel affects your whole general health, mood, energy and well being.

Stand up and walk around the store when trying on shoes. You should have at least a half-inch of space between end of shoe and your longest toe while standing with full weight on your feet. The back of the shoe, however, should fit snugly without any rubbing or slipping up and down that could cause blisters, etc. Be sure and wear the right stockings or socks when trying on shoes.

Width as well as length is important in buying shoes. Move your fingers across top of shoe with your foot in it. A ripple of leather should be evident with a proper fit. Avoid shoes that are tight at the foot's widest point. Do buy shoes that are the proper width for your feet.

Check by feeling the inside of both shoes to make sure there are no stitching ridges, wrinkles, bumps, hard seams or any other protrusions that will rub against your feet and cause blisters or other irritations. Flexible shoe soles are desireable - hold shoe upside down and bend between the sole and heel area to check for some flexibility. Avoid all pointed shoes, boots, etc. that pinch the toes and throw the foot off balance causing corns, bunions, posture problems and health problems

Check these popular shoes on their websites:

- www.ecco.com
- www.rockport.com
- www.newbalance.com
- www.asicstiger.com
- www.mephisto.com
- www.birkenstock.com

Women have four times as many foot problems as men do.

High Heels Can Cause Pain & Wreck Health

Women should wear high heels with caution, and then only for special occasions. Low-heeled shoes are the best choice for day-to-day wear as they keep heels flat to the ground, much like walking barefoot as Mother Nature intended. High heels force the whole body forward, causing the back to curve in, the stomach to protrude and muscles in the legs to shorten. Women's female organs suffer from being tilted and off balance while walking in high heals (*on toes and balls of feet*). This is your body's way of compensating for being thrown off balance, but it can result in mounting aches and pains from your toes to your back and neck.

Tips for Buying the Best Sport Shoes

When you run, your feet hit the ground more than 1,000 times per mile! In aerobics, the weight of your body slams into your soles, which are usually hitting against a concrete or wood-based floor (most gyms have a layer of carpeting down to cushion impact, but unless specially constructed to be spring-loaded the layer under the carpet is generally very hard). Tennis and other racquet sports cause you to twist and turn your feet unnaturally when reaching to return a wayward shot.

So you can see the importance of spending the money to buy a well-made specific sport shoe that is especially designed to be supportive, cushioned in the right places and comfortable for your feet. By wearing the proper sports footwear, you reduce chances of developing overuse injuries such as shin splints, arch strain, blisters and tendonitis.

The ideal sport shoe will not only support your feet, but will provide cushioning to the ankles, knees, hips and back. You can give yourself extra protection by investing in Dr. Scholl's Air-Pillow Comfort Insoles or other foot pads found in your local sport stores, etc. You can cut them to fit perfectly inside any shoe. If you use them regularly, be sure and take a pair with you when trying on future new shoes. This is an inexpensive way to provide additional comfort to any shoe, but particularly walking, running, sport or dancing shoes.

Sports Shoes Buying Check List:

When shopping for sport shoes, use this selection method to make certain you get the best, most comfortable shoes that will fit your body's needs:

- When standing, you should be able to put the width of your index finger between the end of the shoe and your longest toe. This is extremely important, for when the sole hits the ground, the shoe will grab and your foot will slide forward. If the shoes are too short, they will create a jamming, stubbing action on the toes, resulting in sore, swollen toes and can even cause black toenails. (If you have shoes like this, give them to your local thrift store – they might fit someone.)

- While holding the shoe in your hands, flex the sole at the ball of the foot. If the shoe only bends at the arch, there is not enough support, the lack of which could lead to knee pain, a crucial situation for runners and other athletes. The sole should be flexible, yet firm throughout its length.

- Again holding the shoe, squeeze the sides of the heels where they join the sole. This area should be very firm in order to keep your heel supported and eliminate slipping (heel pads are available, if needed). Proper fitting shoes will do away with blisters and calluses, while reducing problems in the ankles, shins and knees.

Sports Shoes Composed of Following Parts:

- **The Outsole:** This part contacts the ground and takes the most abuse. It should provide traction as well as shock absorption. The wafflebottom soles were designed for cross-country running because they provide a gripping property and stability in wet grass or dirt. They are not suitable for cement or wood floors.

- **The Midsole:** This is between the outsole and the insole. It is usually a cushioning material such as ethylene vinyl acetate (EVA), which not only provides cushioning but also stability in a shoe.

- **The Insole:** This is the inner lining of the shoe, usually removable, designed to cushion the foot. Many models come with arch support inserts.

- **Heel Counter:** This is the rigid shoe material that encompasses the heel. Most shoes have internal heel counters but some have an external heel counter or stabilizer made of hard plastic at the base of the heel counter to help control excessive heel rotation. This is an important part of any quality running shoe.
- **The Upper:** The upper part is no longer limited to leather or canvas. Today, uppers are often made of a combination of materials, including nylon mesh for breathability and pigskin for support.
- **Lacing:** There are many lacing systems available, including speed laces that use hooks instead of eyelets and convenient (*easy to do*) velcro backed strap fasteners.

Here are Shoes for Different Sports:

- **Aerobic Shoes** should be lightweight enough for dance moves, but durable. The outsole needs to be more flexible and a stiff heel counter helps prevent overuse syndromes. Those with weak ankles should consider hightops.

- **Tennis Shoes** tend to be heavier to provide more stable support for the side to side movements required for tennis. Leather uppers are popular for support and durability. A rigid heel counter is again recommended.

- **Basketball Shoes** also need to be heavier than running shoes for additional support and durable enough to withstand the punishment of the sport. The midsole should be firmer than running shoes for more ankle support and provide shock absorption. A stiff heel counter, hightops and cushioned innersoles are all recommended to reduce the chance of ankle injuries.

- **Running Shoes** should have at least a half-inch of midsole cushion to absorb shock and should also have a stiff heel counter. Make sure when fitting that your shoe has a roomy toe box. Allow at least a half-inch extra toe length in all shoes. During runs, often the feet can swell by a full shoe size or more.

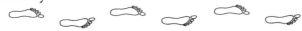

The seat of knowledge is in the head; of wisdom, in the heart.
We are sure to judge wrong if we do not feel right. – William Hazlit

Runners Need Good Shoes

If you are a runner who weighs more than 180 pounds, you should make extra sure you purchase a shoe designed to carry the weight. Most running shoes are designed for the light to midweight runner (no more than 175 pounds). The vertical impact on the shoe increases quickly for heavier runners and can lead to more injuries. Ask your sports shoe salesman for shoes specifically designed for heavyweight runners. Also consider adding your own insole (such as the Spenco or Dr. Scholl's) to help dissipate the ground impact.

Avoid the temptation to buy cheap running shoes, or to use shoes not designed for running. Sports physicians note that one potential consequence is excessive, repetitive trauma to the sensory nerve passing along the inside of the heel. The nerve sheath begins to enlarge into a heel neuroma and pressure on the nerve fibers produces a mild burning or tingling sensation at first, that later develops into pain. If the runner continues despite the pain, it can lead to constant heel pain that requires surgery. This condition is most likely to occur in people who have excessive pronation.

Many people use running shoes for walking shoes, but serious walkers should purchase a shoe made for walking. The foot operates much differently in walking than in running. There is a smoother heel-toe transition, and the impact on the heel is much less for walkers. A beveled heel is recommended. The outsole should be extremely flexible. Some additional midsole cushioning is built in to propel the walker off the midfoot and onto the ball of the foot. The heel counter doesn't have to be as stiff. Uppers should be breathable with pigskin reinforcement for lateral movement.

Wearing the right shoes for your sport helps guarantee a better performance with pain free feet in the sport and activity of your choice. Remember, take care of your feet and they will take care of you for your entire lifetime!

Studies have revealed that fat stored in the body's "spare tire" around the waist increases the risk for diabetes, heart disease and shortens the lifespan!

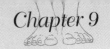

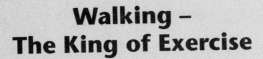

Chapter 9

Walking –
The King of Exercise

About 2,400 years ago, Hippocrates said, "Walking is man's best medicine." Recently, the consensus of those at the National Institute of Health was that walking is the most efficient form of exercise and the only one you can wisely follow safely all the years of your life.

There is nothing as pleasurable as walking. When taking a walk, open your eyes wide and keep your mind receptive to what is around you: see new flowers blooming, hear birds singing. To enjoy the various seasons of Mother Nature are so rewarding to watch because each season has its own individual beauty!

If our feet are *killing* us, all the joys of walking are gone. Many people forego the pleasure of walking because their feet cry out in pain with every step. Use this Course of Foot Care to find new joy in taking walks.

Walking is one of the best overall exercises to keep your feet and entire body happy, fit and healthy. It is the king of exercises and can be enjoyed alone or with a group of people. It is something everyone at all ages can participate in: children, students, working people, retired persons and seniors. There is always a way to incorporate walking into your lifestyle; walking to school, the store, to work, etc. Park a little distance away from where you are going and walk the rest of the way.

Walking utilizes our 260 bones, 640 muscles and 70,000 miles of circulatory channels. Every part of the body benefits from walking! Barring disabling injuries or conditions, walking comes as naturally to us as breathing. A regular walking program will increase lung capacity and actually improve your breathing patterns while improving your circulation and health!

The Medical Journal Circulation reports that people who don't make efforts to exercise regularly face the same dangerous risk of heart disease as people who smoke a pack of cigarettes daily.

Benefits of Walking are Abundant

The muscles of the feet, calves, thighs, buttocks and abdomen all work when you walk. The oxygen your body needs to function properly is distributed more effectively. The heart works harder, sending blood coursing through your veins to improve your entire circulation. Even low or moderate-intensity walking can offer many important cardiovascular benefits, according to medical researchers. Regular walking: 3 to 4 times a week for 30 to 60 minutes, depending on intensity, can help normalize cholesterol, blood pressure, elimination and also fights osteoporosis.

Walking also reduces anxiety and tension and aids in weight loss. There are 3,500 calories in a pound of fat. If an overweight person walks just 20 minutes a day and does not change their eating habits, they can start losing weight.

Other benefits include the strengthening and toning of muscles, weight control and ridding the body of toxins through perspiration. A regular exercise program such as walking also has a tremendously positive effect on mental attitude. Just the act of getting out and doing something physical is, in itself, a mood elevator. The increase of blood circulation in the brain lifts the spirits, calms you down and makes you feel more self-confident. There are also chemical reactions caused by brisk walking that increase the level of endorphins, which are vital chemicals in the body that make us feel good!

Walking is an exercise that needs no gym, natural medicine that requires no prescription, weight control without diet, a cosmetic not sold in a drugstore. It is the tranquilizer without a pill, the therapy without a psychoanalyst, the fountain of youth that is no legend. A walk is a healthy mini-vacation that does not cost a cent. So, it's easy to see that there is nothing to lose and everything to gain by investing in a good pair of walking shoes and going for a healthy fun walk.

Just as the body flourishes on a healthy diet, our joy flourishes with mother nature's beauty. – Thomas Kinkade, visit www.thomaskinkade.com

---

Enter – or perhaps re-enter – the brave new world of wellness through exercise, natural remedies, alternative therapies, meditation and positive thinking.
– Monica Skrypczak

The Bragg Philosophy of Walking

Walk naturally with head high, chest up, feeling physically elated. Carry yourself proudly, straight, erect and with an easy action of swinging arms. Go at your own stride and with your spirit free. If the world of Mother Nature fails to interest you, turn to the inner world of the spirit. As you walk, your body ceases to matter and you become as near to being a poet as ever you will be, each step bringing you inspiration.

Enjoy Your Walk – Leisure or Brisk

There are two different kinds of walks you can take, the leisurely stroll and the brisk, disciplined walk designed for maximum isotonic (heart and circulatory) benefit. If you haven't been involved in an exercise program for a while, walking is the perfect way to get back into the exercise habit. It helps condition you for other activities such as aerobics, jogging or competitive sports like tennis, cycling and swimming and in winter skiing.

As with any new activity undertaken, it's important to start slowly and to know your limits. If you are over 35 or have been inactive because of illness, etc, ask your health professional to give you a treadmill stress test. This helps determine whether your heart can tolerate continuous high-speed walking or leisurely walking.

An old Spanish proverb says, "Walk 'til the blood appears in the cheeks, but not the sweat on the brow," is good wise advice for novice walkers. Here are some guidelines on proper walking techniques. What you don't want to do is to walk slumped over with toes pointed outward, arms flailing and feet landing flatfooted. Your head and back should be erect and shoulders relaxed with arms swinging. The buttocks should be tucked in slightly, even when walking. The toes should be pointed straight ahead when walking and remember your big toes are your foot captains! When walking your eyes should be looking at least 4 yards ahead. Walking with straight posture, *and lifting up your chest*, gives the walker a higher center of gravity and a longer stride.

The average person takes approximately 8,000 steps per day.

The arms should swing naturally in an arc about the shoulder. For a faster walking style, bend the arms 90° at the elbows so the arms can match the quicker leg movements. *(Some walkers like to use hand weights.)* Exhale and inhale breathing deeply and rhythmically, counting one breath for each one, two, or more steps. Soon, this super breathing style becomes second nature. Do read the Bragg Breathing Book for more breathing exercises. See chapters detailed on web: *www.bragg.com*

When smooth striding, the heel should land first. Strive to eliminate any up-and-down or side-to-side movements and concentrate on smooth fluid forward movements for a flowing comfortable walking gait.

On your first four days out, simply walk what is comfortable for you. One sports expert recommends beginning with 15-25 minutes of walking three times a week. (Don't forget that you also have to walk back unless you arrange for a ride at the other end, which is a little self-defeating if done beyond the first week.) On the fifth day, increase your distance by 25%. Five days later, increase the new distance by another 25% and so on.

Start out with a walking pace that doesn't create a strain. Distance is more important than speed. It's advisable to wait until you've been walking regularly for at least a month before you pick up the pace, and then only speed up to a pace that is comfortable for you. The United States Army recommends a pace of 3 miles per hour. This is based on the length of stride and standard height of the average American male. Most women walkers, despite a shorter average height, can handle this pace without strain, once they've reached a level of good overall fitness and health conditioning.

The important thing, however, is to find a stride speed that feels good to you! If you find, using a pedometer, that you're walking less than 3 mph but feel you're getting a good workout without overexerting yourself, then this is the pace you should maintain. At the 3 mph rate, one mile should take you about 20 minutes - a pleasant time that passes quickly once you get into the spirit of the walk and enjoy the scenery and quietness.

Be Faithful with Your Walking Program

Once you start your walking program, it's extremely important to stick with it if you're looking for long-term health and fitness benefits! How do you keep yourself in the program? The best way is to schedule your daily exercise just as you do your other daily activities: your daily shower at 7 a.m., lunch break at noon, etc. Plan to walk from, say, 6:30 to 7:00 a.m. before your shower most mornings. Before you drift off to sleep at night, tell yourself that the first thing you're going to do after getting up is go for your walk. Soon it will become as much a habit as brushing your teeth and tongue. It will start your day off in a natural, invigorating way that will give you a healthy glow and happy frame of mind until bedtime into dreamland, that is a guarantee!

Another option is to take your daily exercise walk on your lunch hour, a wonderful way to escape the afternoon monotony. The increase in circulation, plus the beauty of the scenery, will invariably refresh you and cause you to return to work ready to go. Contrast this to the lack of energy shown by people who have spent their lunch hour snoozing, smoking, drinking or eating heavy foods. If you're hungry, stop in a park, etc. on your walk, relax and enjoy an impromptu picnic of some organic fruit, raw veggies, trail mix, nuts or some soy yogurt, then continue on your walk.

You can also walk when you get off work, to unwind and cleanse your mind and body of the stresses of the day. Pick a natural, beautiful place. Within 20 minutes, you will feel like a renewed person. Plus you will be working up a genuine earned appetite for dinner!

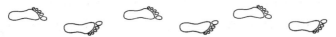

I have the wisdom of my years and the youthfulness of The Bragg Healthy Lifestyle and I never act or feel my calendar years! I feel ageless! Then why shouldn't you? Start living this Bragg Healthy Way today! – Patricia Bragg

I never suspected that I would have to learn how to live – that there were specific disciplines and ways of seeing the world that I had to master before I could awaken to a simple, healthy, happy, uncomplicated life.
– Dan Millman - A Bragg fan since Stanford University coaching days.

Walking Energizes and Refreshes

Make your walking a priority and stick with it. If you have a hard time getting yourself going, try the buddy system. Make arrangements with a family member, friend or neighbor to call each other on a rotating basis. Having someone to encourage and support your efforts definitely helps. It also gives you the responsibility of helping them. Besides, both of you will benefit from having someone to talk to about how great your life is becoming on the walk to make those miles slip away!

Another way to keep your interest level high is to vary the route you take. This can be done on a daily, weekly or strictly random basis. Make a deal with yourself to notice 10 new sights on your walk each day. This will not be difficult. Plan to make each walk an exciting adventure! Make the most of your walking! Enjoy the tranquility that comes with appreciating Mother Nature and God's wonders. As you walk, pray, meditate or sing, *Health, Strength, Youth, Vitality, Joy, Peace* and *Fulfillment* for *Eternity!* Sing or say it silently, shout it out or make up a song to keep time with your stride. Just make sure the message is positive and reinforcing! Make it part of your walking program. It will reward you in many ways beyond happy feet and a healthy body!

When You Are Ready for Jogging - Prepare

Once you have hit 5 to 6 miles of walking at a steady pace, you may feel inclined to start jogging. By this time your muscles, lungs, heart and mind will have become conditioned for a more strenuous workout. But, again, be sure to check with your doctor if you have any concerns about overloading your body and its systems.

Work into jogging gradually. Walk at maximum speed for five minutes and then jog for 60 seconds at a slow pace. Then walk again, followed by another 60 second jog. Alternate jogging and walking about five times. Do this for a week and then gradually increase your jogging.

To desire to be healthy is part of being healthy. – Seneca

As soon as you feel confident that you're not putting undue stress on your heart, feet or leg muscles, add another 10 to 20 seconds and decrease your walking time by the same amount. Generally, it is advised by sports experts that you wait one to two weeks between these changes.

Within a few months, you should be able to do light jogging non-stop for 20 to 30 minutes and you may also want to add more speed to your workout. But remember, your body is the best judge of your capabilities! Trust it and be aware of any signs that may be an indication that you are overdoing it. A few "trouble signals" to be aware of are extreme short-windedness, dizziness, sharp pains in any muscles, joints or bones, cramps, chest pain or a sudden feeling of fatigue.

Take Precautions to Avoid Injuries

If you experience any of the aforementioned "trouble signals," stop jogging immediately and rest or resume walking at a reduced pace. Sometimes the symptom is a temporary warning that you are creating stress on certain body areas. By slowing down, many aches, pains and reactions will simply disappear. However, if any of the symptoms persist or become uncomfortable, it's wise to see your doctor before starting to jog again.

You would not consider entering a professional auto race without having a finely tuned, specially designed car under you to insure peak performance. The same principle applies to jogging. You need those finely tuned, specially designed shoes to maximize your efforts and reduce the possibility of any breakdown of your precious body's equipment. Of course, if you are able to jog barefoot on soft sand or grass, giving you a fabulously free feeling, do not hesitate to do so. Running barefoot on a natural surface is one of life's greatest pleasures! But if you must wear jogging shoes, wear good ones your feet like!

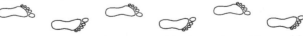

Trans fats such as margarine, solid vegetable shortening, chips and fast food french fries, are so bad for you because they are made with artificial fat that the body can't recognize and therefore has trouble burning, so it's absorbed instead to cause clogging problems. – Dr. Jack Scaff, famous cardiologist

Safe Walking and Jogging is Important

Do not scrimp. Buy top-quality shoes. Refer back to the *Tips on Buying Sport Shoes* Section. A good shoe with proper support and cushioning will prevent such jogger's ailments as shin splints, bone spurs in the ankles and heels, small bone fractures and other impact related problems. (See previous chapter for more info on runner's ailments and their prevention.)

Another way to avoid injury is to jog only on surfaces such as beaches, dirt trails and short grass. Go barefoot when possible. If not possible, wear the proper shoes. Whenever possible, avoid concrete sidewalks, bike paths or hard-packed tracks on high school or college premises.

There is one other very good reason not to jog on city sidewalks. Toxic automobile fumes or smog will do your body more harm than the jogging does it good! We've all seen joggers, intent upon improving their health, running along a busy thoroughfare and deep breathing in the toxins spewed out by passing cars, trucks and bus exhaust. Maximize your efforts by jogging in a park, field or other natural environments.

If you live in an area with cold and snowy winters, check with the local YMCA, high school, college or health and sport clubs to see if they have an indoor track. Be sure to find out if the track is built on a *spring-loaded* floor or is carpeted to reduce injury. Many of these organizations have certain times set aside for joggers and for a small fee you should be able to continue your exercise program even in the dead of winter.

An exciting piece of equipment now available in most sporting good stores and department stores is a home-size trampoline. This is another excellent alternative for working out through the colder months. A great workout without risk of foot or leg injuries, as the trampoline absorbs up to 85% of impact from your body weight. We have one in the house and keep one in the garden.

See web: www.urbanrebounding.com – www.askwaltstollmd.com.

104

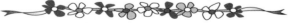

The American diet is overloaded with too much food and the harmful fats that raise blood cholestrol levels that can cause fatal heart disease!

The Optimum Stretch

You can easily incur sprains, pulled muscles or tendonitis by hitting your stride without first warming up. A pre-jog walk will help loosen the body and prepare you for greater exertion. However, the best and most effective warmup is simple, slow stretching. It's the safest way to elongate the muscles and increase flexibility.

Stretching expert Bob Anderson, a Bragg follower for years, recommends stretching for 8 to 10 minutes before and after jogging. He also suggests that you feel free to take short stretching breaks at any time during the jog, walk or run when you experience soreness or tension. For more info see Anderson's web and book: *www.stretching.com*

A good stretch should be done smoothly and slowly, without any jerking or bouncing motions. Stretch to the point where you feel a slight tension on the muscles and hold for 10 seconds. The longer you hold the stretch, the less tension you should feel. Never *push* the stretch or put prolonged tension on the muscles.

Return to your starting position, relax for a few seconds and then stretch again, moving into the stretch a bit further so you experience slight tension. Hold for 10 seconds. If the tension does not diminish, ease off to a more comfortable position. Stretching should never be a strain! If you find that at first you can not fully reach a position or can only stay in the position for a short time, do not worry. You will soon notice an increase in flexibility by stretching regularly.

It is not necessary to limit your stretching to before and after a workout. In fact, it is a method of relaxation that can be incorporated into your daily life: at work, in the morning to limber up, after a long meeting or anytime you feel like it! Don't forget to exercise and stretch toes and feet to keep them strong and flexible.

The preservation of health is a duty. Few seem conscious that there is such a thing as physical morality. – Herbert Spencer

---

I used to say, "I sure hope things will change." Then, I learned that the only way things are going to change for me is when I change! – Jim Rohn

Barefoot Promotes Happy, Healthy Feet

Although you can stretch out your toes, ankles and feet while wearing shoes, it is far more beneficial and relaxing to enjoy the ritual of stretching while barefoot!

By now, you are aware of our philosophy of keeping your feet unhampered by shoes and socks as much as possible. Encourage friends and family to learn to enjoy going barefoot. Create a house rule that no one can wear shoes in your home! The Japanese have followed this practice for centuries. It is not only healthful, but you will find the carpets need to be vacuumed less frequently when shoes are removed upon entering the house.

If some friends seem a bit reluctant at first to go barefoot in your house, provide slippers for them to wear. Keep a supply of inexpensive paper slippers at the front door (available in hospital supply houses or better drugstores). Before long, you will find that your friends will look forward to slipping off their shoes and they will probably bring along a pair of socks (tennis socks are ideal) or scuffs of their own when they visit. This is another way you can share your new-found knowledge about building strong, sturdy, healthy, happy feet!

THE HEALTH LAWS OF LIFE

Man's body was created according to the laws of chemistry and physics, which are the Creator's own laws. They never vary. His law is written upon every nerve, muscle and every faculty that has been entrusted to us. These laws govern the cells, tissues and organs of the body as they carry on their various busy functions around the clock. They operate largely through the complex network of nerves that run throughout the body. They act through the central nervous system, from which nerve impulses originate, and through the autonomic nervous system, that part of the network not under the direct control of the will. It's important we protect our body from wrong living, actions and deeds to help us be perfect in all ways.
– Henry W. Vollmer, M.D.

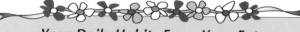

Your Daily Habits Form Your Future
Habits can be good or bad, healthy or unhealthy, rewarding or unrewarding! The right or wrong habits, decisions, actions, words and deeds are up to you! Wisely choose your habits, as habits and lifestyles can make or break your life!
– Patricia Bragg, N.D., Ph.D., Health Crusader

Chapter 10

The Healing Properties of Herbs

Herbal, Holistic and Dietary Remedies For Foot and Joint Ailments

"You are what you eat, drink, breathe, think, say and do!
"What is on the plate today, we become tomorrow."
– Patricia Bragg, N.D., Ph.D.

With these two wise Bragg epithets in mind we may deduce that we can address imbalances and dysfunctions within our body by looking at what we put into it. Whereas damage may already have been done due to years of bad dietary habits, the body has incredible recuperative powers if only we give it a chance to use them.

For example, in dietary terms there is a strong direct correspondence between certain foods and beverages and gout. As we know, gout is caused by a build-up of uric acid crystals in the joints of the foot. Certain foods (generally protein rich foods) are high in a compound called purine which raises uric acid levels. Therefore limiting or eliminating altogether the intake of these foods will help lower the frequency and intensity of gout attacks. Cut out red meats, bouillon and gravies, liver, kidney, sweetbreads and other organ meats, coffee, refined sugar and white-flour products, alcohol, spices, scallops, anchovies, rich, greasy and oily foods in general.

What to eat: Brown rice, celery, tomatoes, seaweed, cherries, blueberries, bananas, kale, cabbage, parsley and all leafy green vegetables. What to drink: distilled water, vegetable and fruit juices - especially cherry, carrot, parsley and celery juice. See herbs pages 109-116 for effective remedies for existing gout and joint symptoms.

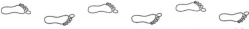

You cannot have a foot problem without having that problem reflected in other parts throughout your body. – Dr. Elizabeth H. Roberts, Podiatrist

Of all knowledge, that is most worth having is knowledge about health. The first requisite of a good life is to be healthy. – Herbert Spencer

Remedies for Athlete's Foot

For athlete's foot a variety of herbal remedies can be taken both orally and applied to the area of infection itself (see herbs opposite). Having some helpings of acidolphus or soy yogurt each day creates good bacteria which combats the unwanted bad bacteria that causes athlete's foot.

Here are some natural treatments which can be applied directly to athlete's foot: After thoroughly washing the feet with warm soapy water, rinsing and drying, massage in garlic oil 2 to 3 times daily. Onion juice may be applied in the same way until symptoms reduce. Alternatively, soak feet twice daily in a solution of Bragg's Organic Apple Cider Vinegar and 70% warm water. (*Also read The Bragg Apple Cider Vinegar Book for more info*). Black walnut tincture is another well tried remedy to be applied externally frequently until you see improvement.

Finally, try soaking your feet in black tea. Add 2-3 tea bags to pot of boiling water. Cool mixture, and soak feet for half-hour. Tannic acid in black tea kills some of the fungus, also provides soothing relief for painful feet.

To combat foot odor try this wonderful foot soak: Pour two quarts of hot water into foot bowl and add a half cup of Bragg's Organic Apple Cider Vinegar and 10 drops of tea tree essential oil and mix thoroughly. Soak feet in this solution for 15-30 minutes, and allow to dry in air for at least 5 minutes.

To overcome smelly shoes make mixture of 3 Tbsps. ground dried sage leaves and 3 Tbsps. of baking soda. Sprinkle 1 Tbsp. of mixture into shoes at night, shake around entire inside of shoes and leave overnight. Wear shoes the following day with mixture still inside, and remove and replace with fresh mixture nightly.

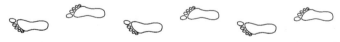

Sad Facts – each year, over 86,000 amputations, especially of the foot, are performed among people with diabetes. Over 15.7 million people in the United States alone have diabetes, which represents 6% of the population.
– American Podiatric Medical Association, www.apma.org

Herbs and Their Healing Properties to Relieve Foot Ailments, Gout and Arthritis

Mother Nature has strewn the earth with a myriad of plants and herbs with miraculous, but often underestimated healing powers, yet still mankind has chosen to go down the road of creating artificial chemicals to try and cure his ills. It's important to understand that we are part of nature, and that our own natural pharmacy is all around us in the countryside, forests and oceans.

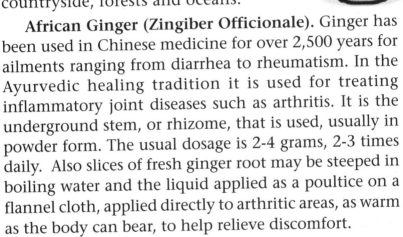

African Ginger (Zingiber Officionale). Ginger has been used in Chinese medicine for over 2,500 years for ailments ranging from diarrhea to rheumatism. In the Ayurvedic healing tradition it is used for treating inflammatory joint diseases such as arthritis. It is the underground stem, or rhizome, that is used, usually in powder form. The usual dosage is 2-4 grams, 2-3 times daily. Also slices of fresh ginger root may be steeped in boiling water and the liquid applied as a poultice on a flannel cloth, applied directly to arthritic areas, as warm as the body can bear, to help relieve discomfort.

Birch Leaf (Betula Alba). An infusion of Birch Leaf can be prepared for flushing out uric acid from joints and for alleviating arthritic pain. Add 1 Tbsp. fresh leaves to 2 cup of boiling water. Cool, and take twice per day.

Boswellia (Boswellia Serrata). This is a resin gleaned from a tree which proliferates in India. Many studies have shown that Boswellia, which is potent in the treatment of osteoarthritis and rheumatoid arthritis. About 150 mgs. three times daily of the standardized extract of the gum oleoresin of Boswellia is the usual dosage. It is recommended you continue this for 8 to 12 weeks.

Briar Hip, Blueberry, etc. (Rosa Canina, Vaccinium Myrtillus). All the berries in the blue/black family have potent diuretic properties and flush out uric acid from joints.

Healthy organic foods and herbs have abundance of potential life energy!

Buchu (Barosma Betulina). A Buchu herbal infusion may be taken 3 times per day, adding one teaspoon of the fresh leaves (2 tsps. if dried leaves are used) to a cup of boiling water, allowing to brew for a good 5 minutes, then strain. This bush, a native of South Africa, has been used to treat so many ailments that it has been described by medical botanists as being *'the Buchu plant is used to treat every disease which afflicts mankind.'*

Burdock (Arctium Lappa). Burdock is a biennial plant found near fences and roadsides. The root of Burdock is effective in the treatment of gout and rheumatism. In Japan, the roots and leaf stalks are boiled twice then eaten. In the west the traditional dosage is 2-4 ml of burdock root tincture per day. For the dried root in capsule form, 1-2 grams may be taken three times per day.

Marigold (Calendula Officianalis). Commonly 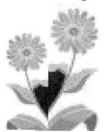 known as Marigold, Calendula may be taken in infusion form 3 times per day with the boiling water being added to 4 cup fresh flower petals, or 2 tsps of dried flowers. Allow to infuse for 5 minutes, then strain. Drink 3 times per day. The tea may also be allowed to get cold and then applied directly to infected area using a soft cloth. This flower with anti-fungal and antibacterial properties has been used to treat other skin ailments such as eczema and skin ulcerations. The flowers have been used as a food coloring and for flavoring soups, vegetables and salads.

Marigolds

Cayenne (Capsicum Frutescens). Cayenne contains a resinous substance known as Capsaicin which provides pain relief by acting on sensory nerves. The effect is temporary, but effective, in providing relief from arthritic pain. It is the fruit that proffers the capsaicin, which is normally administered in cream form. Its counter-irritant action - diverting attention from the original source of pain by depleting neurotransmitters sent out by nerves to the problem area - lends its potency in treating joint pain. Cayenne is usually applied in cream form, although an infusion can be prepared using 2 to 1 tsp. of powder to a cup of boiling water. To keep your feet warm sprinkle 2 Tbsps. of cayenne pepper into a pair of woolen socks. Put on a pair of white cotton socks, and over these the woolen socks with the cayenne pepper. Your feet will stay as warm as toast.

Celery (Apium Graveolens). Both the crushed seeds and the juice of the celery (stalks, leaves) plant are potent in the treatment of rheumatoid arthritis and gout due to their diuretic properties. To make an infusion, pour a cup of boiling water over 1-2 tsps. of freshly crushed seeds and let stand for 10-15 minutes. Take 3 times per day. For juice, use a juicer to extract fresh juice. Take 1-2 Tbsps. 2 or 3 times per day one hour before meals.

Cherry (Prunus Serotina). Having organic cherry concentrated juice, dried cherries or eating a 2 pound of cherries on a daily basis has proven effective in the lowering of uric acid levels and the prevention of gout attacks. Cherries are rich in anthocyanidins (flavenoids with anti-inflammatory properties), which also help to neutralize excess acidity - in particular uric acid.

Clove (Caryophyllus Aromaticus). In Chinese medicine cloves have long been used to treat athlete's foot and other fungal infections, and medieval German herbalists used them as a gout treatment. Cloves have antimicrobial properties effective against fungi and bacteria. Apply cotton wool dipped in clove oil to the affected area. Or prepare an infusion of the 1tsp clove powder to 1 cup of boiling water. Drink 3 times per day.

Coix (Coicis Lachryma-jobi). Also known as Job's Tears, the seeds of this herb may be used to treat rheumatic and arthritic symptoms. To infuse add 1-3 ounces to a cup of boiling water. Alternatively prepare a porridge of 3 grams of Coix and Cinnamon-twig tea with brown rice.

Follow the steps of the Godly instead, and stay on the right path, for good men enjoy life to the full. – Proverbs 2:20-21

Wear proper fitting footwear at all times as there are over 280 different foot ailments that can be suffered. – American Podiatric Medical Association

Comfrey (Symphytum Officinale). For an effective treatment to reduce pain and inflammation during pronounced arthritic attacks, make a sap of 1 tsp comfrey powder or 3 tsp tincture to 3 Tbsp Bragg Organic Apple Cider Vinegar. Soak cloth or gauze in mixture and apply to needed area of ankle, foot, etc. or any area of joint or muscle problems. Leave on overnight, repeating for several nights. Wrap area in soaked gauze and then saran wrap and after a clean, dry cloth. Leave on overnight. Remove upon awakening in the morning. When the pain has reduced somewhat, massage St. John's Wort Oil into the area before going to bed. This simple mixture helps promotes inner healing.

Daisy (Bellis Perennis). The Daisy flowers have a reputation for being beneficial against arthritic and rheumatic symptoms. To infuse, pour a cup of boiling water onto 1 tsp. of dried daisies and allow to brew for 10 minutes. Take 3 to 4 times daily.

Evening Primrose (Oenothffa Bionnis). Evening primrose oil is beneficial for the treatment of rheumatoid arthritis, diabetes and helps relieve menopausal symptoms. The oil contains gamma linolenic acid (GLA) which promotes the production of prostaglandin E1 (PGE1), an important hormone-like substance. Conditions such as diabetes impede the body's natural production of GLA. 3,000 - 6,000 mgs of evening primrose oil daily is recommended which provides 270-360 mgs of GLA.

Gotu Kola (Centella Asiatica). The leaves of this perennial plant native to India, Sri Lanka and other tropical countries have properties which make them an effective herbal combatant of athlete's foot. Prepare an infusion by adding boiling water to 4 cup of fresh leaves or 2 tsps. of the dried variety. To anul the bitter taste somewhat you may add honey or lemon. Let stand for 5 minutes, strain and drink. You may also apply as a wet compress bandage and cover with plastic wrap, then cover foot with cotton sock.

Gravel Root (Eupatorium Purpureum). The rhizome and the root may be used to prepare an infusion to treat rheumatoid arthritis and gout. Pour 1 cup of boiling water over 1 tsp. of the fresh herb and allow to infuse for 10 minutes. Drink 3 times per day.

Guaiacum (Guaiacum Officinale). Guaia, the resin from a tree native to Central and South America, Mexico and the West Indies, is useful in the treatment of gout and the prevention of its recurrence, also to alleviate symptoms of rheumatoid arthritis. To make an infusion pour boiling water over 1 tsp. of the wood chips and allow to stand for 15 to 20 minutes. This infusion you may drink 3 times per day.

Guggul (Commiphora Mukul). Guggul is a gum resin obtained from a small tree (also known as the Mukul Myrrh Tree), which is native to India and certain Arabic countries. The resin is used in Ayurvedic medicine for the treatment of inflammatory conditions such as rheumatoid arthritis and gout. It is normally taken as a herbal supplement in tablet form.

Gymnema (Gymnema Sylvestre). This climbing plant that is found in Central and Southern India has been used for the treatment of diabetes for over 2,000 years. The leaves have the effect of lowering blood sugar and raising insulin levels. 400 mgs per day for periods of up to 18 or 20 months have been recommended. Alternatively 2 to 4 grams of leaf powder may be used.

Horsetail (Equisetum Arvense). This healing herb is renowned for its usefulness in treating arthritis and gout. An infusion taken 3 times daily will help eliminate uric acid build up. Horsetail contains Potassium, 15 types of bioflavinoids and is rich in silicates. This natural silicon content is the active anti-arthritic agent. Pour boiling water over 2 Tsps of the dried Horsetail, allowing to infuse for 15 to 20 minutes. 3 2 ounces of Horsetail added to bathwater makes a soothing bath to alleviate arthritic pains.

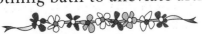

Kelp (Fucus Vesiculosus). This sea vegetable is also known as Bladderwrack, this seaweed is reputed to alleviate symptoms of rheumatoid arthritis both by taking internally in infusion form, and using externally, by applying the same topically to inflamed joints. Pour cup boiling water onto 2 tsps. dried (*or powder*) kelp. Take 3 times daily. (*We sprinkle kelp granules over our food*).

Marsh Clover (Menyanthes Trifoliata). Also known as Bogbean, Bog Myrtle and Marsh Trefoil, the leaves of this herb have diuretic properties and are renowned for their beneficial action against osteo-arthritis and rheumatoid arthritis. For an infusion pour a cup of boiling water onto 1-2 tsps. of the dried leaves. Allow to steep for 10-15 minutes. The infusion may be taken 3 times per day.

Parsley (Petroselinum Crispum). An infusion of Parsley can be prepared to help flush out uric acid from tissues and joints and to help alleviate

arthritic pain. Pour 1 cup of boiling water on to 1-2 tsps. of fresh leaves or root and infuse for about 5-10 minutes. in a closed container. Take twice per day. Parsley should not be used during pregnancy or if you have a kidney infection.

Sarsaparilla (Ichnocarpus Fruitescens). Used widely in Ayurvedic medicine, Sarsaparilla root is excellent for gout, and a poultice of the infusion of the root and leaves may be applied topically to painful, arthritic joints. Pour 1 cup of boiling water over 1 tsp. dried sarsaparilla powder. Drink twice daily or apply direct to affected area.

Stinging Nettle (Urtica Dioica). Drinking a cup of stinging nettle tea 3 times per day for 3 weeks will help eliminate uric acid build up in the joints. Stinging nettles strengthen the whole body, are an excellent general detoxifier and are particularly effective in the treatment of arthritis. Pour boiling water onto 1-3 teaspoons of the dried herb and allow to infuse for 10-15 minutes.

Visit this great website on herbs: www.herbs.org

Tea Tree (Melaleuca Alternifolia). In 1770, Captain James Cook came across a grove of trees with aromatic leaves from which he and his party made tea. It was not until much later (after the first world war) that the real medicinal properties of Tea Tree Oil were investigated. Among the essential oils, tea tree has few rivals with regards to its anti-infectious properties. It was discovered that the oil of the tea tree is 12 times stronger than carbolic acid as an antiseptic bactericide. Tea tree is powerfully antibiotic and extremely beneficial to the human body and immune system. Tea tree oil is potent in the treatment and prevention of a number of bacterial, viral and fungal infections.

To treat Athlete's foot, apply a few drops of the oil to the infected area 4 times per day until it appears that the problem has cleared. Continue to apply for two to four weeks afterwards to make sure every trace of the fungi has disappeared. (Also review pages 14-16, 18, 79-80, 108).

Tumeric (Curcuma Longa). Tumeric's anti-inflammatory properties make it potent in treating arthritis. Recommended dose is 400 mgs, 3 times daily.

White Poplar (Populus Tremuloides). This herb has the reputation of being effective in the treatment of rheumatoid arthritis, especially in reducing discomfort when there is much pain and swelling. May also be used for arthritis in conjunction with other herbs such as celery, bogbean and black cohosh. Put 1-2 tsps. of the dried bark in a cup of water, bring to a boil and allow to infuse for 10-15 minutes. May be drunk 3 times per day.

Wild Yam (Dioscorea Villosa). The dried roots of this herb are excellent for the treatment of rheumatoid arthritis, especially for soothing and subduing acute periods of intense inflammation. Put 1-2 tsps. of the dried root into a cup of water, bring to a boil and allow to simmer for 10-15 minutes. Should be taken 3 times per day.

Lavender helps you relax. Before drying off in the shower, place 3 drops of essential lavender oil on a damp sponge or washcloth and gently rub it over your body. The soothing, relaxing active agents in the lavender oil will enter your body through your skin and nose.

Willow (Salix Alba). The bark from this tree native to central and southern Europe and North America has analgesic, anti-inflammatory and pain relieving qualities, which prove effective in the treatment of osteoarthritis and rheumatoid arthritis. An infusion can be prepared by boiling 1-2 grams of bark in 200ml of water for 10 minutes. This can be drunk up to 5 times per day.

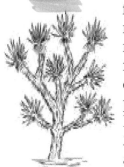

Yucca (Yucca Schidigera). This desert tree is useful for the treatment of osteoarthritis and rheumatoid arthritis. A study has revealed that saponins (soapy textured fluids) from the yucca stop the release of toxins from the intestines, which prevent regular formation of cartilage. For arthritis it is recommended to take 2 capsules of yucca twice per day on an empty stomach.

It's Important To Remember The Following When Using Herbal Remedies:

Pregnant women and diabetics should consult a herb specialist or their health doctor before embarking on a course of herbal therapy. It's also important to take into consideration that some herbs when taken alongside conventional prescription medication may cause some reactions - again advice should be sought.

For more herbal info visit these websites:

- www.wellnet.ca/herbsa-c.htm
- www.herbs.org
- www.herbscancure.com/arthritis.htm
- www.holistic-online.com
- www.lacetoleather.com/athletesfoot.html
- www.herbsfirst.com/discriptions/athletesfootpg.html

80% of all foot problems can be attributed to ill-fitting footwear.
– Dr. William A. Rossi, Podiatrist and constultant to the footwear industry

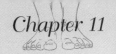
Foot Reflexology

Foot reflexology is a form of therapy that involves manipulating specific areas, or zones of the body. These zones are directly linked to the reflex points of all the various organs and nerves in the body. The most sensitive zones are found in the toes, soles, arches and ankles of the feet.

Foot reflexology is an effective way to energize and rebalance the corresponding organs. It is also extremely beneficial in the reduction and even the elimination of pain in the body. In addition, it relieves nervous tension, slows the ageing process, increases circulation and can help you free yourself from illness.

Sound like a miracle? It is. It is a miracle that you can easily learn and use to promote a more healthful, vital way of living for yourself, your family and friends. Everyone, from infants to older people, can benefit from this simple reflexology technique. The accompanying charts are provided to help you learn the basic reflex points. For more info, see web: *www.reflexology-usa.net*

We are proud that Eunice D. Ingram, a pioneer in the reflexology field in America, was a Bragg follower. She became a student during a Bragg Health Crusade in Florida as a young girl and was a faithful follower of our Bragg Healthy Lifestyle all her life. In fact, she said it was Paul Bragg that led her to the study of foot reflexology to help her grandmothers aching feet.

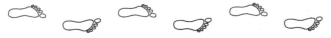

Recent studies revealed that fat stored in the body's "spare tire" around the waist increases risk for diabetes, heart disease and other serious health problems! Shocking fact: the bigger the waistline, the shorter the lifespan!

The nation badly needs to go on a healthy diet. It should do something drastic about excessive, unattractive, life-threatening fat. It should get rid of it in the quickest, safest possible way and this is by fasting, exercise and living a healthy lifestyle. – Allan Cott, M.D., Author, *Fasting As a Way of Life*

117

How Does Reflexology Work?

Running between each organ, nerve and gland are channels or currents which send vitalizing energy through our bodies in much the same way that electrical wires carry electrical currents. Often, a channel becomes blocked because of illness, injury or nervous tension. Through reflexology and massage, we can open up these blockages and allow the energy to flow freely again.

For example, a winter cold may produce symptoms such as a headache, sore throat, earache and even a stiff neck. By applying pressure to the corresponding zones on the feet in a systematic way, you will be able to relieve these painful and irritating symptoms. This will work whether the problem is a cold, congestion, backache, digestive ailment, poor circulation, insomnia or depression.

Reflexology is Effective Self-Therapy:

1. The feet are easily accessible for reflexologists and great for self-reflexology and massage treatments.

2. The pressure points are simple to find since the feet are tender from being covered and encased most of the time in socks and shoes. In addition, there is little fat or muscle in the feet to interfere with therapeutic effects of massage. It's also possible to feel the buildup of toxic crystal deposits which indicate problems in corresponding body areas.

3. A short cut to learning reflexology is looking at charts that show which body parts correspond to certain areas of the feet. This eliminates the need for advanced anatomy studies.

4. The miracle feet are literally and symbolically our connection with the earth. Because of this, they are especially receptive to the energy which carries us forward each day, and to enhancing that energy.

5. We know that happy pain-free feet are healthy feet. In order to take us through a lifetime, it's important to pamper and protect our feet. Reflexology and foot massages also help improve your general health.

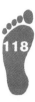

Reflexology – Pressure Foot Points

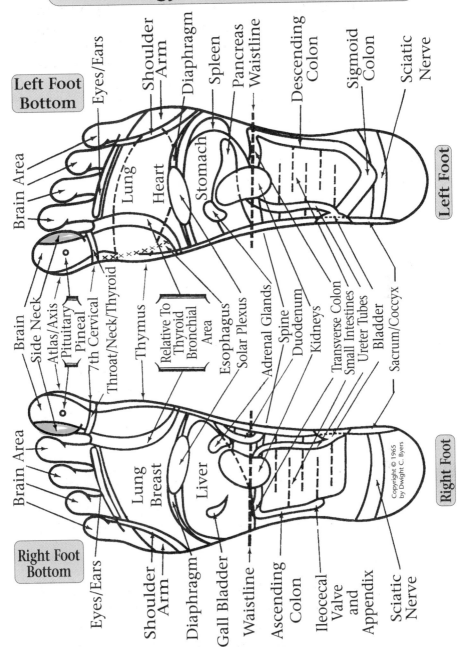

REFLEXOLOGY AND ZONE THERAPY

Founded by Eunice Ingham, author of *The Story The Feet Can Tell,* who was inspired by a Bragg Health Crusade when she was 17. Reflexology helps the body by removing crystalline deposits from meridians (nerve endings) of the feet through deep pressure massage. It helps activate body's flow of healthy energy by dislodging any collected deposits around the nerve endings. (Charts reprinted with permission by Eunice Ingham's nephew Dwight Byers.)
Visit their great website: reflexology-usa.net

Reflexology – Pressure Foot Points

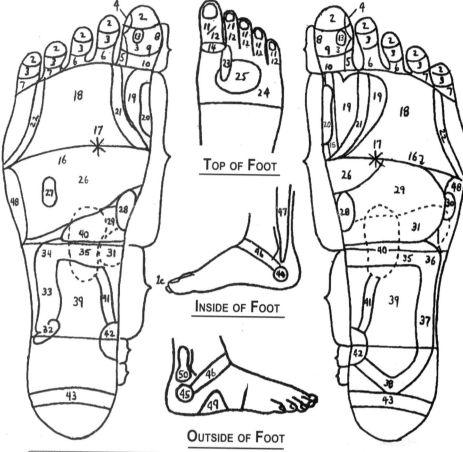

TOP OF FOOT

INSIDE OF FOOT

OUTSIDE OF FOOT

Right Foot

Left Foot

1. Spine   a. Cervical,
   b. Thoracic c.Lumbar,
   d. Sacrum, e. Coccyx
2. Brain
3. Sinuses
4. Temple
5. Side of Neck
6. Eye, Inner Ear
7. Outer Ear
8. Nose
9. Mouth
10. Throat, Thyroid
11. Jaw (top)
12. Teeth / Gums, (top)
13. Pituitary / Pineal
14. Thyroid / (top), Throat
16. Diaphram
17. Solar Plexus

18. Lung
19. Heart
20. Thymus
21. Bronchial Tube
22. Shoulder
23. Lymph Drain (top)
24. Ribs / Upper Back (top)
25. Breast / Mammary
    Glands (top)
26. Liver
27. Gall Bladder
28. Adrenal
29. Stomach
30. Spleen
31. Pancreas (dotted line)
32. Beocecal Valve (Appendix)
33. Ascending Colon
34. Hepatic Flexure

35. Transverse Colon
36. Splenic Flexure
37. Descending Colon
38. Sogmoid Colon / Flexure
39. Small Intestines
40. Kidney (dotted line)
41. Ureter Tube
42. Bladder / Sacroiliac Joint
43. Sciatic
44. Uterus / Prostate
45. Ovary / Teste
46. Falopian Tube / Lymph Drain
47. Chronic Area
48. Arm / Hand
49. Hip / Knee / Leg
50. Hip / Siatic

120

Reprinted with permission By: Jane Kerns, **Reflexology Center of Honolulu, Hawaii**

Reflexology – Pressure Hand Points

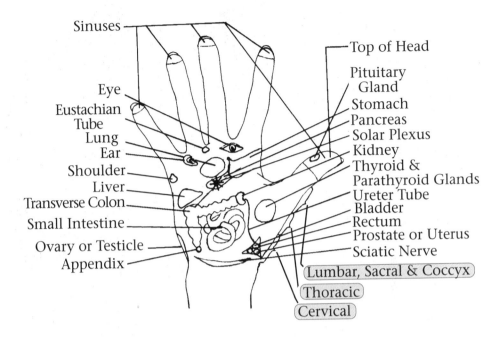

Sinuses

Top of Head

Pituitary Gland

Eye

Stomach

Eustachian Tube

Pancreas

Lung

Solar Plexus

Ear

Kidney

Shoulder

Thyroid & Parathyroid Glands

Liver

Ureter Tube

Transverse Colon

Bladder

Small Intestine

Rectum

Ovary or Testicle

Prostate or Uterus

Appendix

Sciatic Nerve

Lumbar, Sacral & Coccyx

Thoracic

Cervical

Acupoints of the Ear

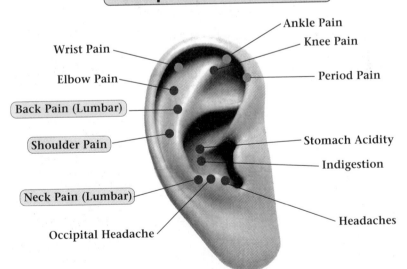

Ankle Pain

Knee Pain

Wrist Pain

Period Pain

Elbow Pain

Back Pain (Lumbar)

Shoulder Pain

Stomach Acidity

Indigestion

Neck Pain (Lumbar)

Headaches

Occipital Headache

Apply strong pressure using index finger and thumb (place thumb at back of ear). Squeeze point for about two minutes, then massage (We do this nightly). You can repeat this throughout the day whenever convenient (acupressure ear points are bilateral – same on both ears). Ear points respond well to acupressure and can be combined with other body acupressure points or used by themselves.

121

Acupoints of the Spine

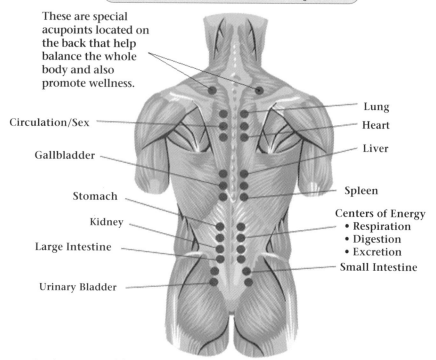

These are special acupoints located on the back that help balance the whole body and also promote wellness.

Circulation/Sex

Gallbladder

Stomach

Kidney

Large Intestine

Urinary Bladder

Lung

Heart

Liver

Spleen

Centers of Energy
• Respiration
• Digestion
• Excretion

Small Intestine

Design created by David Carmos, Ph.D. from *The Acupoint Book* and *You're Never Too Old To Become Young* by David Carmos, Ph.D. and Shawn Miller, D.C. (See Web: *www.perfecthealthnow.com*)

What is Acupressure?

Acupressure Potent Points is an ancient healing art that uses the fingers to press key local points on the skin's surface to stimulate the body's natural self-curative inner healing abilities. When these points are pressed, they release muscular tension reaching also to the body's trigger points to promote healthier blood circulation and increase the vital life force to aid healing. Acupressure is the most effective method for self-treatment of tension-related ailments by using the power and sensitivity of the touch of the human hand. See web: *acupressure.com*

How Acupressure Can Help Relieve Pain

One of the popular alternative therapies available to help relieve back pain is acupressure, which is often described as *acupuncture without needles*. Acupressure is a system of massage that promotes the life energy, stimulating meridian points whether needles or fingers are used.

Acupressure You Can Do Yourself

Foremost among the advantages of acupressure's healing touch is that it's safe to do on yourself and others – even if you've never done it before – just follow the instructions and go gently and slowly. There are no side effects from drugs and the only equipment needed are your own two hands. You can practice acupressure therapy anytime, anywhere on friends, family and yourself! The acupressure points are areas on the body that are sensitive to the body's bioelectrical impulses. When you stimulate these points, it triggers the release of natural endorphins. As a result, pain is blocked and the flow of blood and oxygen to the affected area is increased. This causes the muscles to relax and promotes healing.

Besides relieving pain, the acupressure can help rebalance the body by dissolving the tensions and stresses that keep the body from functioning smoothly and which inhibit the immune system. Troublemaking tension tends to concentrate around acupressure points. Along with Acupressure, you can use a combination of the self-help methods given in this book that can help improve your overall health and you will feel more alive, healthy, and in harmony with your life. *With our love and blessings,*

Patricia and *Paul C. Bragg*

Morning Resolve To Start Your Day

I will this day live a simple, sincere and serene life; repelling promptly every thought of impurity, discontent, anxiety, discouragement and fear. I will cultivate health, cheerfulness, happiness, charity and the love of brotherhood; exercising economy in expenditure, generosity in giving, carefulness in conversation and diligence in appointed service. I pledge fidelity to every trust and a childlike faith in God. In particular, I will be faithful in those habits of prayer, study, work, nutrition, physical exercise, deep breathing and good posture. I shall fast for a 24 hour period each week, eat only healthy foods and get sufficient sleep each night. I will make every effort to improve myself physically, mentally, emotionally and spiritually every day.

Morning Prayer used by Patricia Bragg and her father, Paul C. Bragg

123

Healing Through Reflexology & Acupressure

Reflexologists worldwide have thousands of case histories which testify to the many miraculous healing capabilities of these forms of massage. Although reflexology is not considered a cure for such conditions as terminal illness, broken bones or certain neurological diseases, it has proven extremely effective in treating health problems and even to emotional disorder and infertility. See web: *www.footreflexology.com*

It would be impossible to describe here in detail all the benefits to be derived from this type of therapy. If you are considering using foot reflexology as a healing technique, we recommend you read as many books on the subject as you can find. There are also courses available through community colleges and specialized massage schools which will provide the licensing necessary to practice this art as a professional.

Setting the Stage For Massage

There is no question that massage, foot reflexology and acupressure will help promote general well-being and the recovery of sick organs and gland in a safe and more natural way. It's also the most relaxing and caring treatment you can do for someone, including yourself and even pets.

Knowledge of the reflex points is of vital importance. Also, an understanding of the basic strokes and techniques used will make the massage a positive and enjoyable experience for both parties involved – the person giving the massage and the recipient. The beauty of massage and foot reflexology is that the more you learn and understand, the greater the health benefits become. Not only will you be helping others, you will be increasing your personal fulfillment through sharing your talent. The act of sharing and giving is its own reward.

A good way to familiarize yourself with reflex points and techniques is to start on your own feet. One rule to remember is to keep the first foot reflexology and massage treatments to about 20 minutes, as the immediate effect of ridding clogged channels of toxins may cause a reaction, such as slight feelings of wooziness or nausea. Begin with a short session, wait one day and then work the feet again.

Message calms the nervous system, allowing better communications between the organs and the body to operate more effectively!

Relaxation is The Key For Best Treatment

The first step in self foot reflexology is to find the most comfortable, relaxing position to work in. If you are working on your feet, try sitting in a chair, your bed or even the floor. The location does not matter; the important thing is that you find a comfortable sitting or resting position which permits you to rest the foot you will be massaging on the opposite thigh.

When working on someone else's feet, have them lie down or sit in a chair opposite you and rest the foot being treated in your lap. Some reflexologists find it very soothing to have their patients soak the other foot in a basin of warm vinegar-water to stimulate circulation.

The key to successful foot reflexology is relaxation of both the practitioner and the patient. If you are tense or feeling ill, it would be best to postpone the treatment if possible, because your tension will be transferred to the patient's body and you can actually draw energy away from the other person. That will reduce, if not eliminate, the benefits of the treatment. If necessary, get into a relaxed mood with a calming backdrop of candles, flowers and soft music. Environmental sounds, available in music stores such as ocean waves, waterfalls and singing birds, etc., can be very calming!

If you find you must talk at any time, perhaps to explain what you are doing, speak in soft, hushed tones to maintain the relaxing peaceful mood. Another wonderful way to relax your patient is to wash the feet prior to starting the massage. Many civilizations have used this as a way of welcoming and honoring guests. The host would perform this ritual to show respect and also to soothe the spiritual energy of arriving friends.

Soak the feet for 10 to 15 minutes in warm vinegar-water. It can be plain water, or enhanced with herbal tea bags and a few drops of scented massage oil such as clove, cinnamon or peppermint. Brush the feet vigorously with

---

Relaxation techniques are very important benefits to the body's general health and cardiovascular system. Such techniques as sitting quietly, deep breathing, meditation and ignoring distracting thoughts can bring down blood pressure and are free of side effects. – Harvard Health Letter

a cloth or a loofah sponge while feet are still in the water. Dry thoroughly and then start your massage. The feet will be invigorated and sensitive at this point and your patient will be fully relaxed to enjoy maximum pleasure and benefit from the foot and ankle massage.

Make sure your hands are warm before placing them on the feet. This can be done by rubbing them briskly or holding them under warm water. (You should always wash your hands before and after giving a foot and also a body massage for obvious hygienic reasons.)

Be gentle when you first make contact with the feet. This is extremely important for you in order to get a feeling for the overall attitude of the person you massage. Are they tense or relaxed? The initial gentleness will also serve to make the recipient feel more comfortable about you working on their feet. If the person seems tense, just hold one foot for a minute or so to gain their confidence. Then start with a slow, light stroking to get the blood flowing.

Gradually work your way along the sole, over and in between the toes, up the sides of the foot and around to the heels and ankles. Ask the person to tell you if any areas seem more sensitive than others. By studying foot charts, you will be able to pinpoint and pay extra attention to any sensitive problem areas.

A Variety of Massage Techniques to Use

Here are some different massage techniques and strokes you can use to open up blocked channels and encourage new flow of rejuvenating energy;

- **Kneading** – This is just like working bread dough and can be used to work on large areas of the foot, such as the under-arch. It is very powerful as a means of stimulating muscle reflex points.

- **Vibration** – Put one finger or the heel of the hand on a specific point and move it back and forth in a rapid, gentle motion and then move on to other points. This creates an immediate energy surge to the corresponding organ, nerve or gland.

126

The human body has one ability not possessed by any machine – the body has the ability to repair itself. – George W. Crile

- **Acupressure** – Use the thumb or knuckle to apply steady and firm pressure to a specific reflex point. Acupressure is excellent for overall toning and for the repairing of corresponding organs.

- **Basic Massage** – Using all the fingers and the thumbs, work quickly and lightly with a release/grip/release/stroke/release/grip action. The result will be very relaxing, yet energizing.

- **Rubbing** – Just as it implies, you rub the feet between your two hands to stimulate blood flow throughout the feet and the entire body.

- **Wringing** – Imagine you are wringing out a wet washcloth, using both hands, twist each hand in opposite directions, going up and down the foot. This motion is one of the most relaxing and it's advisable to have your patient rest after their treatment.

You will, as you study and practice foot reflexology, add other strokes. Some are in books you can read on the subject. Others you will discover for yourself. When you try a new technique, a simple way to gauge its effectiveness is to ask the person you are massaging if it feels good. If so, keep it in your routine.

Each person has a different "pain threshold". That is, some may be able to take a strong, steady pressure to a specific area, say the tips of the toes. Yet another may find it unbearable to have you touch the feet with anything other than a gentle rubbing stroke. Assure your patients that you will honor their request for harder or softer pressure. If they have this sense of trust in you they will receive greater benefit from the foot treatment.

Foot reflexology is a wonderful, natural way to improve the body's functions and increase your overall health and happiness. It's an art that is easily learned.

The study of foot reflexology will provide you with a method of massage you can share with others, and what greater gift is there than the gift of self? It's a special talent that will add to your joy of living. This alone will make you a happier and more fulfilled person.

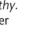

Self discipline is your golden key; without it, you can't be happy and healthy.
– Maxwell Maltz, M.D. author *Psycho-Cybernetics* and a Bragg follower

Take Time for 12 Things

1. Take time to **Work** –
   it is the price of success.
2. Take time to **Think** –
   it is the source of power.
3. Take time to **Play** –
   it is the secret of youth.
4. Take time to **Read** –
   it is the foundation of knowledge.
5. Take time to **Worship** –
   it is the highway of reverence and
   washes the dust of earth from our eyes.
6. Take time to **Help and Enjoy Friends** –
   it is the source of happiness.
7. Take time to **Love and Share**–
   it is the one sacrament of life.
8. Take time to **Dream** –
   it hitches the soul to the stars.
9. Take time to **Laugh** –
   it is the singing that helps life's loads.
10. Take time for **Beauty** –
    it is everywhere in nature.
11. Take time for **Health** –
    it is the true wealth and treasure of life.
12. Take time to **Plan** –
    it is the secret of being able to have time
    for the first 11 things.

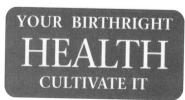

YOUR BIRTHRIGHT
HEALTH
CULTIVATE IT

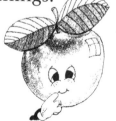

Have an

Apple

Healthy Life!

128

*Teach me Thy way O Lord, and
lead me in a simple plain path.* – Psalms 27:11

Chapter 12

Questions and Answers

Q. *What's the difference between an Orthopedist and a Podiatrist?*

A. Orthopedists are medical doctors (M.D.'s) who have specialized in the diagnosis and treatment of bone and joint ailments. Some may focus on either hands or feet, and are authorized to perform surgery if needed.

Podiatrists are college graduates who have gone on to complete four additional years at one of six U.S. podiatry colleges and have been awarded a Doctor of Podiatric Medicine (D.P.M.) degree. About half of the graduating podiatrists complete additional residency in foot surgery. See web: www.apma.org

Podiatrists specialize in diseases and injuries of the feet and may be consulted for all basic foot ailments such as corns, calluses and ingrown toenails. Podiatrists may treat you directly or refer you to other specialized physicians such as orthopedists when necessary.

Q. *What are Orthotics?*

A. Orthotics are supports that are inserted into shoes to correct imbalances and defects of standing, walking and running. Up until a decade or so ago, Orthotics were usually custom-made by a podiatrist and could be quite costly. Now Orthotics are relatively inexpensive.

Orthotics may help correct defects such as pronation, the turning inward of the ankles as a person walks or runs. This puts pressure on the inside of the foot and can lead to flattened arches or even bunions. An Orthotic can build up the inside of the shoe so that pressure is even and redistributed toward the outside. Supination, the turning outward of the foot at the ankle while walking or running, can also be helped by an Orthotic. The proper Orthotic builds

---

Caring hands have healing life-force energy. All ages, even babies to family pets thrive on daily soothing, loving, healing, touching and massages. Everyone benefits from healing massages and treatments!
– Patricia Bragg, N.D., Ph.D., Health Crusader

up the outside of the shoe and forces the foot inward to even out the weight distribution. People with one leg longer than the other can also benefit from an Orthotic in the shoe of the shorter leg. Check web: *www.goodfeet.com*

Of course, for problems caused by weak ankles or poor posture, Orthotics provide only temporary relief, and the Bragg Foot Exercises should be done faithfully to strengthen the weak areas and will help correct the defects.

Q. How early should I allow my daughter to begin ballet lessons? I've heard permanent foot damage can be done if she starts ballet toe dancing too young.

A. Ballet lessons for grace and posture may begin at any age, but toe on pointwork should not be taught until bones and muscles are sufficiently developed to prevent physical deformity! We do not endorse toe ballet dancing.

Q. I dried my rain-soaked shoes in front of a heater, and now they're stiff. What did I do wrong?

A. Wet shoes should never be quick-dried by artificial heat. This will cause them not only to crack, but to shrink. The only proper procedure is to stuff them with newspaper or tissue and allow them to dry slowly and naturally.

Q. I've heard recently that lasers are being used for foot operations. Is this true?

A. Yes, it is. In recent years, carbon dioxide lasers have been employed to remove warts, to treat severe ingrown toenails, and for other purposes. The advantage of using a laser is that the beam of light is very focused, so surrounding tissue is hardly affected by the operation. Also, lasers sterilize and seal blood vessels as they cut, so there is less bleeding, reduced chance of infection and a shorter recovery time!

Q. Why do high heels make women's legs look good?

A. Because high heels shorten the gastrocnemius and soleus muscles in the back of the leg. This may add shape to the calf, but it does so at the health expense of muscle flexibility and body function. In other words, the calf muscles may become permanently shortened, thereby

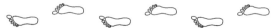

It's magnificent to live long if one keeps healthy, active and fit. – Harry Fosdick

ruining proper posture and movement. Do not make a habit of wearing high heels! If you desire shapely legs, do Bragg foot and leg exercises and go for daily walks. Also see more exercises on the web: www.bragg.com

Q. My son was born with flat feet. How will this limit him?

A. It used to be thought that flat feet, the lack of an arch at the instep, would cause difficulty in walking. The Army rejected many men on this basis during the First World War, until it was shown that men with congenital flat feet were least likely to suffer foot pain during long marches. So your son, happily, won't experience any limitation in his walking ability. About 5% of the population have flat feet, the same amount that show the opposite, an unusually high arch.

Q. I've been told that men and women develop different kinds of running injuries. True or false?

A. True. New research indicates women experience more problems with ankles and hips, men with feet and knees. This is probably due to the differing pelvic structures. However, all the various running ailments can be found all too frequently in both sexes, because too many runners do not pay attention to the pain messages from their bodies – sad facts – often until it is too late! Also, unnatural surfaces like roads and sidewalks tend to produce more injuries. Always wear appropriate shoes on these hard surfaces and whenever possible, walk or run on natural surfaces such as dirt, grass, or sand. Barefoot running is ideal and remember to stretch first.

Q. What are shin splints?

A. Shin splints is a blanket term for a variety of injuries to the front of the lower leg, mostly caused by overuse and excess pounding of feet and legs on hard surfaces. It is an inflammation of the muscle, tendon or bone of the lower leg. Pain is never gain! If the fronts of your legs become tender during or after walking or running, it's best to rest them and analyze the problem.

If exercise could be packed into a pill, it would be the single most widely prescribed and beneficial medicine in America. – Robert Butler, M.D.

13

As a rule, shin splints will respond well to symptomatic treatment and do not permanently hamper an athlete's performance. If persistent pain is an ongoing problem, this may call for change in training routines, rest or for the use of orthotics. Pain in the lower leg can also be the result of a stress fracture or compartment syndrome. Determine cause of pain to correct, so it won't continue and happen again!

Shin Splints Prevention Measures

- *Increase the flexibility of the front and back muscles of the leg through regular stretching.*
- *Wear well-fitting shoes with shock-absorbing soles, inner sole padding and stiff heel counters.*
- *Avoid prolonged training on hard surfaces.*
- *Avoid sudden increases in training routines.*

Many sports physicians recommend general treatment measures such as contrast bath treatments. This involves placing lower leg in cold water footbath for 5 minutes, and alternating with hot footbath for 5 minutes, until the half hour treatment is completed. Finish with a cold footsoak to reduce swelling and pain. Some recommend *ace* taping the lower legs to ease pain and provide support. If these measures don't help, a thorough diagnosis is recommended in case the pain is due to a stress fracture or compartment syndrome.

Q. What can I do about excessive foot sweating and the terrible accompanying odor?

A. See a podiatrist promptly. You don't have to bear these embarrassing conditions! Excessive sweating (hyperhidrosis) and odor (bromidrosis) may or may not occur together and can have a number of causes. Two may be faulty foot posture or a toxic, unhealthy diet. Have a check-up, and faithfully follow The Bragg Foot Program.

Q. How do I use herbal oils on the feet? Which of the oils are especially good for massaging the feet?

A. You can either massage a few drops of the oil directly on the foot, or you can use a footbath, which helps heal and rejuvenate your entire system. To make a footbath, either brew a strong herbal tea and use it directly, or add a few drops of oil (see page 14) to warm (not hot) water. Soak feet in footbath for 10 to 15 minutes, keeping the water warm by adding or replacing some from time to time. Then dry the feet well and massage them with a little more oil, if you desire. This procedure is both wonderfully relaxing and very healing.

Some especially good oils and their effects are: camomile, which is stimulating (opposite of the tea) when used as an oil; cayenne, which detoxifies and increases circulation; coriander, which produces warmth, dries oily skin; garlic, which is an antibiotic; geranium, which revives tired skin; lavender, which can reduce swelling in the legs; and clove and cinnamon, antiseptics which are good to finish off with, either singly or mixed. Strong peppermint tea makes a particularly good footbath!

Q. I have seen a person with toenails that were overgrown, pitted and dull. What causes this?

A. For a problem like this, consult a foot doctor. Cause is probably a fungus, much like the athlete's foot fungus, called onychomycosis. If left untreated, the infection may cause the toenails to powder and fall out! This condition was considered incurable, but now it is treated with antifungal agents, but first try Bragg Foot Program.

Q. Can fallen arches be helped by exercise?

A. Yes! See exercises given in Chapter One, which are good to do for all ages, either to correct weaknesses in foot muscles, or to prevent any weakness from developing. Also, often go barefoot on natural surfaces.

Q. I'm on my feet almost all the time at work. After a few hours, I notice my feet are hurting. At the end of the day, they're literally killing me. What can I do?

A. First, buy the most comfortable, natural shoes you can find that are acceptable at your workplace. These days, such shoes are available for almost all occupations and situations. Second, rest your feet whenever possible. Sit down on your breaks and at lunch, and elevate your feet slightly. If possible, remove your shoes and socks, and give your feet a brief massage. Third, do simple foot exercises while you are standing with your feet inside your shoes. Curl your toes, spread them, roll your weight to the insides and then to outside of your feet, rock gently between toes and heels. And finally, when you get home, remove your shoes promptly, wash your feet, massage them, and follow this Bragg Foot Program faithfully! Also often orthotics do help.

Q. *The skin on my feet is very dry. Please help!*

A. You can do several things to alleviate dry skin and the fissures and cracks that often result. Massage in lubricating oils, as described earlier, as part of your daily footcare. Also try Vitamin A, D, E and herbal creams. Check your diet for ample healthful foods and take multi-vitamin-mineral supplements and try Omega 3, flax oil, cod liver oil and drink ample distilled water and other healthy liquids!

Q. *My husband's feet are always cold. Is there any way he can help correct this problem?*

A. Cold feet have a number of causes. In general, coldness in the extremities could be due to lack of exercise, poor circulation, diabetes, malnutrition, injury or even a nervous condition. This coldness can be worsened by smoking cigarettes, drinking alcohol and coffee - one more reason to give up these unhealthy habits! Nicotine and caffeine close down blood vessels and slow your entire circulation! To increase blood flow, regular daily exercise and hot/cold showers help. Also, faithfully take daily vitamin/mineral supplements and reflexology and acupressure treatments work miracles!

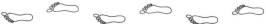

I love to walk among nature's beauty that
adorns our world. – George Santayhana

Staying in shape pays, partly because aerobic activity promotes circulation. If you already have back problems, the right kind of regular exercise will help prevent you from getting more severe pain and further injury.
– Stephen Hochschuler, M.D., Orthopedic Surgeon and Chariman,
Texas Back Institute, Plano, Texas.

Vitamins, minerals, herbs and superfoods optimize healing potential. They offer potent armor to deal with the body-ageing realities of today's environment: mineral depleted soil, strong toxic chemical use, oxygen robbing pollutants, etc. Fortifying your diet with supplements and superfoods strengthens your health and ability to function in a world which makes it tough to be healthy. – Linda Page, N.D., Ph.D., Author of *Healthy Healing* 1(888) 447-2939. Visit Doctor Page's website: www.healthyhealing.com

Q. What causes varicose veins? I think standing all day has something to do with mine. What can I can do to prevent or alleviate this problem?

A. Varicose veins in the legs and feet are caused by faulty valve function in superficial veins. (*It's estimated 25% of women and 15% men worldwide have varicose veins.*) When valves don't work properly, blood backs up and pools instead of circulating freely. This causes veins to swell. The heart, fighting gravity all day, can't muster enough force to send blood back upward. Obesity and even weight gained during pregnancy can increase this tendency (*varicose veins and even hemorroids*), which usually reverses itself within six weeks after childbirth.

This sounds very health serious, and it can be, both cosmetically and in terms of pain and discomfort, but the solution is often easy. Get off your aching feet and elevate them whenever you can! Daily to promote blood drainage lie on your back, put legs up above heart level and gently press hands down legs to get any pooled blood back into circulation. Also, begin an exercise program to strengthen the heart and improve condition of blood vessels (Rutin, CoQ10, Vit.E, Bioflavonoids help). For most people, this should be sufficient to help reverse tendency towards varicose veins. In drastic cases your doctor may recommend stripping (surgical vein removal) or injecting the veins. (*Endovascular Laser is minimally invasive Venacure treatment and it's safer.* www.elvslaser.com*)* It's best to avoid this, so be sensitive to messages your feet, legs and body are sending you, and take action to correct.

Q. I walk and jog a lot, and my Achilles Tendon is often sore. Is there some remedy?

A. Achilles tendonitis is a frequent complaint. It is caused by prolonged or repeated irritation of the tendon, such as occurs in joggers. Each time the Achilles has to lift the body's weight (about 1,500 times a mile for joggers!), it must contract and then stretch. If the tendon is not stretched properly before vigorous walking or running, or if it hasn't had sufficient rest before walking or running again, it becomes sore. If you don't stretch after activity, it may become shortened. Inward rolling of the foot may also contribute to this problem. Check the heels of your walking or running shoes. Is the outside of the back of the sole worn more than the rest? If so, your foot is tilting inward. In fact, checking the wear of your shoes, soles, etc. in general is an excellent way to diagnose posture and gait problems.

To heal Achilles Tendonitis, you must first stay off the feet as much as possible. Do not run until the soreness is gone; swim or ride a bicycle instead. Once you feel back to normal, carefully stretch before walking or running, and don't overdo your activity. Older walkers and runners should take extra care of their Achilles Tendon. Sports physicians recommend only a moderate stretching routine for seniors combined with a half-mile walking warm-up prior to any jogging, running and then another half-mile walking cool down after a run.

To fare well implies partaking of foods which do not disagree with body or mind. Only those who fare well live temperately. – Socrates

---

The treatment of diseases should go to the root cause, and most often it's found in severe dehydration from lack of sufficient distilled water, plus the living of an unhealthy lifestyle!

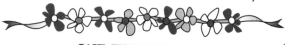

WE THANK THEE

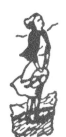

For flowers that bloom about our feet;
For song of bird and hum of bee;
For all things fair we hear or see,
Father in heaven we thank Thee!
For blue of stream and blue of sky;
For pleasant shade of branches high;
For fragrant air and cooling breeze;
For beauty of the blooming trees
Father in heaven we thank Thee!
For mother love and father care,
For brothers strong and sisters fair;
For love at home and here each day;
For guidance lest we go astray,
Father in heaven we thank Thee!
For this new morning with its light;
For rest and shelter of the night;
For health and food, for love and friends;
For every thing His goodness sends
Father in heaven we thank Thee!
- Ralph Waldo Emerson

An excellent stretch for the Achilles tendon is to stand facing a wall, palms against it at shoulder level. Then slowly back your feet outward, leaving your hands against the wall to support your weight. At some point, you'll feel the stretch begin in the tendon. Slowly back outward, taking care to never go beyond gentle stretching, not pain. If you try to stretch too severely, you will make the problem worse, not better. Respect Mother Nature's healing pace, remember healing takes time!

Q. I belong to a health spa where I work out three or four times a week. After each session there, I enjoy taking a sauna and a shower. I'm worried about getting athlete's foot from walking barefoot through the shower room. What can I do to prevent athlete's foot and what should I do if I get it?

A. Although athlete's foot often can be contracted from walking barefoot in gyms, locker rooms and showers, whether or not you get it depends upon your vulnerability to the fungus. If you're susceptible (in other words, have had it before) it's safer to wear slip-on rubber thongs after removing your sport shoes at the health spa.

If you should contract athlete's foot, bathe the feet in a vinegar footbath daily. Dry thoroughly and sprinkle or spray with Desenex or some other special fungus-control product. The inside of the socks should be sprinkled as well. (See pages 14, 18, 79 and 80 for more solutions.) If possible, wear sandals to expose infected foot to the air. If a severe case, affecting entire foot, as well as the toenails, it's advisable to see a foot doctor.

Q. How long must I be off my feet after a sprained ankle?

A. The general consensus is that a person with a mild sprained ankle must not engage in any sports or activities that would put additional strain on the ankles for at least six weeks: it often can take a total of three months before the ankle can be considered back to normal. You might consider swimming as a good substitute for your

Brisk walking is the king of exercise – with walking you discover the beauty of Mother Nature and God, it awakens and softens your soul and life! – Patricia Bragg, N.D., Ph.D., Health Crusader

usual walking or running activities. A mild sprain (involving a stretching but not tearing of a ligament) should be taped for two weeks and treated with hot and cold vinegar soakings.

If a ligament is torn, creating a severe sprain, a walking cast may be required to keep pressure to a minimum. In most cases, the cast will be left on for four to six weeks, followed by a soft elastic bandage for several weeks.

Q. Sometimes when I'm in a phase of heavy jogging, I get worried that I am overdoing it. How will I know when this is a reality worth my concern?

A. Listen to your body! If you have real aches and pains which don't go away within 10 to 15 minutes after you stop jogging, then it's likely you're overextending yourself.

If you've been jogging too much, cut back to shorter distances at a slower pace, or consider cutting back to a walking program for a few weeks to give your body and/or any injured parts a chance to rest. Work out one day, and take the next day off. Continue that pattern until you feel strong again. Invest some time in massage and slow, gentle stretching to warm up sore or injured muscles and help increase the bloodflow to affected area.

Trust your body to let you know when something is wrong and needs more attention and consideration! Remember, walking and running are done to improve your health, not undermine it. Use good sense and moderation in following your Bragg Healthy Lifestyle Program of Exercise . . . after all, it's for a long lifetime of service!

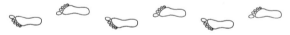

Touch is a primal need, as necessary for growth as food, clothing and shelter. Michelangelo knew this: when he painted God extending a hand toward Adam on the ceiling of the Sistine Chapel, he chose touch to depict the gift of life.
– George H. Colt

Joint and back pains, angina, allergies, asthma, migraines, stomach pains and arthritis may all be symptoms of severe dehydration – can easily be helped by drinking 8 to 10 glasses of pure distilled water daily! Start increasing your water intake today. Be water wise and health safe! – Paul C. Bragg

---

A higher percentage of Americans are obese than Canadians or Britons.
– American Journal of Public Health

Chapter 13

Alternative Health Therapies And Massage Techniques

Try Them – They Work Miracles!

Explore these wonderful natural methods of healing your body. Then choose the best healing techniques for you:

ACUPUNCTURE/ACUPRESSURE Acupuncture directs and rechannels body energy by inserting hair-thin needles (use only disposable needles) at specific points on the body. It's used for pain, backaches, migraines and general health and body dysfunctions. Used in Asia for centuries, acupuncture is safe, virtually painless and has no side effects. **Acupressure** is based on the same principles and uses finger pressure and massage rather than needles. Websites offer info, check them out. Web: *acupuncture.com*

CHIROPRACTIC Chiropractic was founded in Davenport, Iowa in 1885 by Daniel David Palmer. There are now many schools in the U.S., and graduates are joining Health Practitioners in all nations of the world to share healing techniques. Chiropractic is popular, is the largest U.S. healing profession benefitting literally millions. Treatment involves soft tissue, spinal and body adjustment to free the nervous system of interferences with normal body function. Its concern is the functional integrity of the musculoskeletal system. In addition to manual methods, chiropractors use physical therapy modalities, exercise, health and nutritional guidance. Web: *chiropractic.org*

F. MATHIUS ALEXANDER TECHNIQUE These lessons help end improper use of neuromuscular system and bring body posture back into balance. Eliminates psycho-physical interferences, helps release long-held tension, and aids in re-establishing muscle tone. Web: alexandertechnique.com

FELDENKRAIS METHOD Dr. Moshe Feldenkrais founded this in the late 1940s. Lessons lead to improved posture and help create ease and efficiency of movement. A great stress removal method. Web: *feldenkrais.com*

If you have mastered yourself, nature will obey you. – Eliphas Levi

Alternative Health Therapies & Massage Techniques

HOMEOPATHY In the 1800's, Dr. Samuel Hahnemann developed homeopathy. Patients are treated with minute amounts of substances similar to those that cause a particular disease to trigger the body's own defenses. The homeopathic principle is *Like Cures Like*. This safe and nontoxic remedy is the #1 alternative therapy in Europe and Britain because it is inexpensive, seldom has any side effects, and brings fast results. Web: *homeopathyhome.com*

NATUROPATHY Brought to America by pioneer Dr. Benedict Lust, M.D., this treatment uses diet, herbs, homeopathy, fasting, exercise, hydrotherapy, manipulation and sunlight. (Dr. Paul C. Bragg graduated from Dr. Lust's first School of Naturopathy in U.S. Now 6 schools.) Practitioners work with your body to restore health naturally. They reject surgery and drugs except as a last resort. Web: *naturopathics.com*

OSTEOPATHY The first School of Osteopathy was founded in 1892 by Dr. Andrew Taylor Still, M.D. There are now 15 U.S. colleges. Treatment involves soft tissue, spinal and body adjustments that free the nervous system from interferences that can cause illness. Healing by adjustment also includes good nutrition, physical therapies, proper breathing and good posture. Dr. Still's premise: if the body structure is altered or abnormal, then proper body function is altered and can cause pain and illness. Web: *osteopathy.org*

REFLEXOLOGY OR ZONE THERAPY Founded by Eunice Ingham, author of *Stories The Feet Can Tell*, inspired by a Bragg Health Crusade when she was 17. Reflexology helps the body by removing crystalline deposits from reflex areas (nerve endings) of feet and hands through deep pressure massage. Reflexology originated in China, Egypt, American Indians and Kenyans practiced it for centuries. Reflexology activates the body's flow of healing and energy by also dislodging deposits in corresponding areas in the body. Visit Ingham's website: *www.reflexology-usa.net* and *www.reflexology.org*

SKIN BRUSHING daily is wonderful for circulation, toning, cleansing and healing. Use a dry vegetable brush (never nylon) and brush lightly. Helps purify lymph so it's able to detoxify your blood and tissues. Removes old skin cells, uric acid crystals and toxic wastes that come up through skin's pores. Use loofah sponge for variety in shower or tub.

Alternative Health Therapies & Massage Techniques

REIKI A Japanese form of massage that means "Universal Life Energy." Reiki helps the body to detoxify, then re-balance and heal itself. Discovered in the ancient Sutra manuscripts by Dr. Mikso Usui in 1822. Web: *reiki.com*

ROLFING Developed by Ida Rolf in the 1930's in the U.S. Rolfing is also called structural processing and postural release, or structural dynamics. It is based on the concept that distortions (accidents, injuries, falls, etc.) and the effects of gravity on the body cause upsets in the body. Rolfing helps to achieve balance and improved body posture. Methods involve the use of stretching, deep tissue massage, and relaxation techniques to loosen old injuries and break bad movement and posture patterns, which can cause long-term health and body stress. Web: *rolf.org*

TRAGERING Founded by Dr. Milton Trager M.D., who was inspired at age 18 by Paul C. Bragg to become a doctor. It is an experimental learning method that involves gentle shaking and rocking, suggesting a greater letting go, releasing tensions and lengthening of muscles for more body health. Tragering can do miraculous healing where needed in the muscles and the entire body. Web: *trager.com*

WATER THERAPY Soothing detox shower: apply olive oil to skin, alternate hot and cold water. Massage areas while under hot, filtered spray (pages 130-132). Garden hose massage is great in summer. Hot detox tub bath (20 minutes) with cup each of Epsom salts and apple cider vinegar, pulls out toxins by creating an artificial fever cleanse. Web: *nmsnt.org*

MASSAGE & AROMATHERAPY works two ways: the essence (aroma) relaxes, as does the massage. Essential oils are extracted from flowers, leaves, roots, seeds and barks. These are usually massaged into the skin, inhaled or used in a bath for their ability to relax, soothe and heal. The oils, used for centuries to treat numerous ailments, are revitalizing and energizing for the body and mind. Example: Tiger balm, MSM, echinacea and arnica help relieve muscle aches. Avoid skin creams and lotions with mineral oil – it clogs the skin's pores. Use these natural oils for the skin: almond, apricot kernel, avocado, soy, hemp seed and olive oils and mix with aromatic essential oils: rosemary, lavender, rose, jasmine, sandalwood, lemon-balm, etc. –6 oz. oil & 6 drops of an essential oil. Web: *aromatherapy.com* or *frontierherb.com*

141

Alternative Health Therapies & Massage Techniques

MASSAGE – SELF Paul C. Bragg often said, "You can be your own best massage therapist, even if you have only one good hand." Near-miraculous health improvements have been achieved by victims of accidents or strokes in bringing life back to afflicted parts of their own bodies by self-massage and even vibrators. Treatments can be day or night, almost continual. Self-massage also helps achieve relaxation at day's end. Families and friends can learn and exchange massages; it's a wonderful sharing experience. Remember, babies also love and thrive with daily massages, start from birth. Family pets also love the soothing, healing touch of massages. Web: *amtamassage.org*

MASSAGE – SHIATSU Japanese form of health massage that applies pressure from the fingers, hands, elbows and even knees along the same points as acupuncture. Shiatsu has been used in Asia for centuries to relieve pain, common ills, body and muscle stress and aids lymphatic circulation. Web: *www.shiatsu.org*

MASSAGE – SPORTS An important health support system for professional and amateur athletes. Sports massage improves circulation and mobility to injured tissue, enables athletes to recover more rapidly from myofascial injury, reduces muscle soreness and chronic strain patterns. Soft tissues are freed of trigger points and adhesions, thus contributing to improvement of peak neuro-muscular functioning and athletic performance.

MASSAGE – SWEDISH One of the oldest and the most popular and widely used massage techniques. This deep body massage soothes and promotes circulation and is a great way to loosen and relax muscles before and after exercise.

Author's Comment: We have personally sampled many of these alternative therapies. It's estimated that soon America's health care costs will leap over $2 trillion. It's more important than ever to be responsible for our own health! This includes seeking holistic health practitioners who are dedicated to keeping us well by inspiring us to practice prevention! These Alternative Healing Therapies are also popular and getting results: aroma, Ayurvedic, biofeedback, color, guided imagery, herbs, music, meditation, magnets, saunas, tai chi, chi gong, yoga, Pilates, etc. Explore them and be open to improving your earthly temple for a healthy, happier, longer life. **Seek and find the best for your body, mind and soul.** –**Patricia Bragg**

A Personal Message to Our Students
The Body Self-Cleans & Self-Heals When Given A Chance

It is our sincere desire that each one of our readers and students attain this precious super health and enjoy freedom from all nagging, tormenting human ailments. After studying this healthy spine program, you know that most physical problems arise from an unhealthy lifestyle that creates toxins throughout the body. Many of these trouble spots are years old and are mainly concentrated in the intestines, colon and organs.

We have taught you that there is no special diet for any one special ailment! The Bragg Healthy Lifestyle promotes cleansing through the eating of more organic raw fruits and vegetables combined with regular fasting. It is only through progressive cleansing that the human "cesspool" can be banished! We have told you that you will go through healing crises from time to time. During these cleansing times you might have weakness and might become discouraged! This is the time you must have great strength and faith! It is during these crises, when you feel the worst, that you are doing the greatest amount of deep detox cleansing. This is why weaklings, cry-babies and people without will-power and intestinal fortitude fail to follow this perfect Bragg Heathy Lifestyle System of Cleansing and Rejuvenation! Please be strong!

Weaklings want a cure that requires no effort on their part. Mother Nature and your body do not work that way! The average unfortunate sick person thinks of the Lord as a kind and forgiving Father who will allow them to enter the Garden of Eden effortlessly and unpunished for any violation of His and Mother Nature's Laws.

You can create your own Garden of Eden anywhere you live, regardless of climate! All you have to do is to purify the body of its toxic poisons by living a healthy lifestyle. You can reach a stage of health and youthfulness that you never thought was possible! You can feel ageless where your chronological age actually stands still and pathological age will make you younger! When your body is free of deadly toxic material you will reach the physical, mental, emotional and spiritual state that will give you happiness every waking hour as it adds many more youthful, active, joyous years to your life!

143

Say to Yourself: If it is to be - It is up to me!

- ❤ "I will not drink coffee."
- ❤ "I will not use salt."
- ❤ "I will not use tobacco."
- ❤ "I will not over-eat."
- ❤ "I will not drink black tea."
- ❤ "I will not drink sodas."
- ❤ "I will not clog my arteries with saturated fats."
- ❤ "I will not drink alcoholic drinks."

Habits that destroy the health of your body must be broken with a strong willpower! Say to yourself repeatedly and believe it, that your intelligent mind will health captain your body towards super health! Let no person or circumstances break your iron willpower! Let no one brainwash you! You must do your own thinking! You can and will control your own mind, body and health. With inner strength you break bad habits of all kinds!

Coffee and Non-Herbal Teas are Drugs

Coffee is a harmful stimulant to the heart and body! It contains the drug caffeine which makes the heart beat faster and puts it under an undue, unhealthy strain. Coffee also contains tars and acids which are injurious to the heart, blood vessels and other tissues. These same agents are also present in de-caffeinated coffee. Don't drink coffee – it has no nutrients and no vitamins or minerals! Coffee is worthless and harmful to your health! The same goes for non-herbal tea. Don't contaminate your bloodstream with these toxic substances – Black tea contains tannic acid!

Study Shows Cola Drinks Toxic To Body

What do cola drinks contain? Three toxic stimulants and carbonated water! Colas contain caffeine, phosphoric acid and refined white sugar (also some diet colas contain toxic aspartame); all are toxic *empty calories* without any health nutrient value. They also contain carbonated water, which irritates kidneys and liver! Recent study says: *Don't drink colas or any sodas – and don't let your children ruin their health with these drinks! – See www.mercola.com*

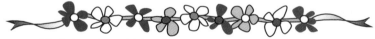

Life is learning which rules to obey and which rules not to obey and the wisdom to tell the difference between the two.

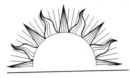 # MY DAILY HEALTH JOURNAL

Today is:____/____/____

I have said my morning resolve and am ready to practice
The Bragg Healthy Lifestyle today and every day.

Yesterday I went to bed at: Today I arose at: Weight:

Today I practiced the No-Heavy Breakfast or No-Breakfast Plan: ☐ yes ☐ no

- **For Breakfast** I drank: Time:
  For Breakfast I ate: Time:

  Supplements:

- **For Lunch** I ate: Time:

  Supplements:

- **For Dinner** I ate: Time:

  Supplements:

- Glasses of Water I Drank and time during Day:
- List Snacks – Kind and When:

- **I took part in these physical activities today:**

Grade each on scale of 1 to 10 (desired optimum health is 10).
- **I rate my day for the following categories:**

  Previous Night's Sleep: Stress/Anxiety:
  Energy Level: Elimination:
  Physical Activity: Health:
  Peacefulness: Accomplishments:
  Happiness: Self-Esteem:

- **General Comments and To Do List:**

Protector of Our Oceans, Sea Life and Waters

Wyland, Famous Whale Wall Artist

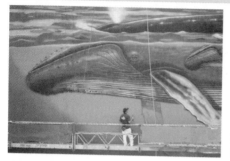

89 Wyland Whale Walls Worldwide

Patricia visits with Wyland at his celebration in Hawaii. As a young man from Michigan, Wyland saw a pair of whales barely 100 yards offshore on his first Pacific Ocean visit. He was so inspired that he devoted the rest of his life to creating art that captures the beauty of these magnificent creatures. It has been more than 25 years since Wyland began painting his landmark marine life murals. Wyland has a passion for whales and the oceans and still has the same sense of unbridled wonder that inspired this young man to make a difference in the world. To date he has painted 89 Walls which is equal to 16,302 feet of murals (3.1 miles). His walls are attractions viewed by over a billion people yearly in 68 cities across the U.S.A. and in these countries: Russia, Germany, China, Spain, Italy, Ireland, Scotland, Poland, India, Africa, Taiwan, Korea, Switzerland, Egypt, Israel, South Africa, England and Norway. These enormous wall paintings include Grey, Minke, Fin, and Blue Whales, Humpbacks and marine life like Sea Turtles and every reef fish imaginable.

Patricia shares in Wylands commitment to the protection and preservation of the world's waters and the abundant life within them. Learn more about Wyland and his great artwork. Visit his website: www.wyland.com

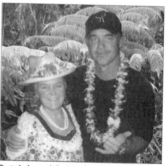

Patricia with Wyland at his 25 year celebration of creating Whale Walls. Wyland follows the Bragg Healthy Lifestyle and has super energy and health.

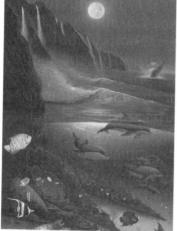

Wyland's "Sacred Waters"

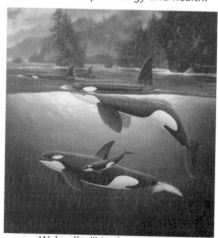

Wyland's "Northern Waters"

With your new awareness, understanding and sincere commitment of how to live The Bragg Healthy Lifestyle – you can now live a longer, healthier life to 120 years!

God bless you and your family and may He give you the strength, the courage and the patience to win your battle to re-enter the Healthy Garden of Eden while you are still living here on Earth with time to enjoy it all!

With Blessings of Health, Peace, Joy and Love,

Paul and *Patricia*

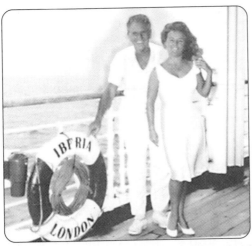

Health Crusaders Paul C. Bragg and daughter Patricia traveled the world spreading health, inspiring millions to renew and revitalize their health.
- 3 John 2
- Genesis 6:3

The Bragg books are written to inspire and guide you to health, fitness and longevity. Remember, the book you don't read won't help. So please read and reread the Bragg Books and live The Bragg Healthy Lifestyle!

I never suspected that I would have to learn how to live – that there were specific disciplines and ways of seeing the world that I had to master before I could awaken to a simple, healthy, happy, uncomplicated life.
– Dan Millman, Author of *The Way of the Peaceful Warrior* www.danmillman.com
A Bragg fan and admirer since Stanford University coaching days.

A truly good book teaches me better than to just read it, I must soon lay it down and commence living in its wisdom. What I began by reading, I must finish by acting! – Henry David Thoreau

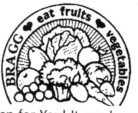

FROM THE AUTHORS

GO ORGANIC

This book was written for You! It can be your passport to the Good Life. We Professional Nutritionists join hands in one common objective – a high standard of health for all and many added years to your life. Scientific Nutrition points the way – Mother Nature's Way – the only lasting way to build a body free of degenerative diseases and premature ageing. This book teaches you how to work with Mother Nature, not against her. Doctors, nurses, and professional care givers who care for the sick try to repair depleted tissues, which too often mend poorly – if at all. Many of them praise the spreading of this message of natural foods and methods for long-lasting health and youthfulness at any age. This book was written to speed the spreading of this tremendous health message.

Statements in this book are recitals of scientific findings, known facts of physiology, biological therapeutics and reference to ancient writings as they are found. Paul C. Bragg faithfully practiced the natural methods of living for over 80 years with highly beneficial results, knowing that they were safe and of great value. His daughter Patricia Bragg worked with him to carry on the Health Crusades. They make no specific claims regarding the effectiveness of these methods for any individual, and assume no obligation for any opinions expressed in this book.

No cure for disease is offered in this book. No foods or diets are offered for the treatment or cure of any specific ailment. Nor is it intended as, or to be used as, literature aimed at promoting any food product. Paul C. Bragg and daughter Patricia express their opinions solely as Public Health Educators and Health Crusaders.

Experts may disagree with some of the statements made in this book, particularly those pertaining to the various nutritional recommendations. However, such statements are considered to be factual, based upon the long-time experience of Paul C. Bragg and Patricia Bragg. If you suspect you have a medical problem, please seek alternative health professionals to help you make the healthiest, wisest and best-informed choices.

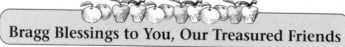

Bragg Blessings to You, Our Treasured Friends

From the Bragg home to your home we share our years of health knowledge – years of living close to God and Mother Nature and what joys of fruitful, radiant, fulfilled living this produces – this my Father and I share with you, your family and loved ones. With Love and Blessings for Health, Peace and Happiness. – Patricia

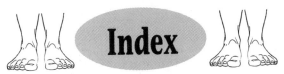

Index

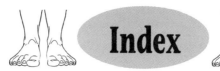

Index

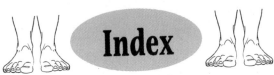

Index

Your life will improve, glow & sparkle with health, if you allow it to!!!

HOW?

If you will take charge, then guide and control your life with health wisdom and love – then you can reach your health goals!!! With love and prayers to you – our health friends.

– Patricia Bragg, N.D., Ph.D., Health Crusader

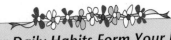

Your Daily Habits Form Your Future

Habits can be wrong, good or bad, healthy or unhealthy, rewarding or unrewarding. The right or wrong habits, decisions, actions, words or deeds . . . are up to you! Wisely choose your habits, as they can make or break your life! – Patricia Bragg

Praises for
Bragg Health Teachings

I was diagnosed with diabetes and had high sugar levels. Within 6 months, I was insulin free. I am healthier now than I have been for the last 15 years. My wife, three young children and I are now all vegetarians and living the Bragg Lifestyle. The results have been amazing. We all thank You.
– Dennis Urbans, Australia

I found your Bragg Books in a health food store. I bought them, read them, gave copies to several friends including my doctor, and I have followed The Bragg Healthy Lifestyle since. I can honestly say that out of all the health books I have read, the Bragg Health Books benefitted me the most!
– Reiner Rothe, Vancouver, B.C. Canada

I love the Bragg Health Books and your Miracle of Fasting. They are so popular and loved in Russia and the Ukraine, for over 20 years. I give thanks for my health and my super energy. I am proud to recently win the Honolulu Marathon in Hawaii with the all-time women's record!
– Lyubov Morgunova, Moscow, Russia

I give thanks to pioneer health crusaders Paul Bragg and daughter Patricia for their long years of dedicated service spreading health and fitness worldwide. It has made a difference in my Life and millions of others worldwide.
– Pat Robertson, Host "700 Club"

The Bragg Books – Healthy Lifestyle, Fasting, Vinegar, and now the Water and Nerve Book are printed in my country, Bulgaria! The Books get great applause by the public and the critics – Three of your books are now on the best seller list! People adore you and want you to come to Bulgaria! Special Greetings from 8 million Bulgarians.
– Syetoslav Iliev, Scorpio Publishing, Bulgaria

The results were miraculous! I got rid of a constant cold, and I feel so good and healthy again.
– Nestor R. Villagra, Toronto, Ontario, Canada

Praises for
Bragg Health Teachings

Rock and roll health is better than rock and roll wealth. Thanks to Bragg, the road ain't a drag anymore. We thank the Braggs for super smooth going and success on our recent whirlwind 20 city tour of England.
– David Polemeni, Boy's Town Band, NJ

I've known the wonderful Bragg Health Books for over 25 years. They are a blessing to me and my family and to all who read them to help make this a healthier world.
– Pastor Mike MacIntosh,
Horizon Christian Fellowship, San Diego, CA

When I was younger (working around asbestos) I inhaled asbestos fibers of which the doctors tell me there is no way to clear it up and no cure. I was not feeling well and my chest hurt. A friend I play golf with here in Santa Barbara, CA., introduced me to your Bragg Organic Apple Cider Vinegar Cocktail. I drink it 3 times a day and also use it over my salads. I am now feeling very healthy and strong! What a blessing. I feel 100% better; It's helping me clean out my asbestos fibers. Thanks to my friend, and to you for such a great product and your vinegar book on all the ways to use your healthy vinegar. I will continue to use and enjoy your health products.
– Al Escalera, Santa Barbara, CA

I read your book on uses for Bragg Organic Apple Cider Vinegar and am now taking it daily. After passing on the book to my mom, she too started using your vinegar and found that the pain in her shoulder that had been waking her up at nights for years has vanished. Thank you.
– Catherine Cox, Toronto, Ontario, Canada

I just read your wonderful book The Bragg Healthy Lifestyle which I heard of through a friend. This book is a great benefit to my health and life and will make wonderful gifts for my friends. Thank you. – Delphine, Singapore

BRAGG HEALTH BOOKS ARE GIFTS FOR LIFE

Gen. 6:3   3 John 2

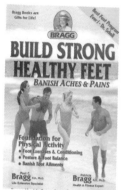

BUILD STRONG HEALTHY FEET
BANISH ACHES & PAINS

Learn how to banish aches & pains. Read about Reflexology, Acupressure and much more. Almost all of us are born with perfect feet. It's the abuse millions give their feet that makes them go limping into adulthood crying, *My aching feet are killing me!*

The Bragg Foot Program is the best ever written. I thank Bragg Books and their wisdom for my long active, healthy life.

0–87790–077–9 – $8.95   **– Dr. Scholl**
Pioneer Foot Doctor

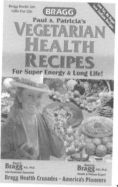

VEGETARIAN HEALTH RECIPES
For Super Energy & Long Life!

Enjoy the worlds finest health recipes for super health and high energy that you and your family will love. Fast and easy to prepare – 100's of delicious healthy recipes enjoyed by millions worldwide.

This book shows how to eat right with nutritious recipes to maintain the body's health and fitness.

0–87790–046–9 – $9.95   **– Henry Hoegerman, M.D.**

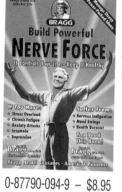

Build Powerful NERVE FORCE
It Controls Your Life – Keep It Healthy

Millions of healthy, happy followers have learned to control and increase their Vital Nerve Force Energy - the Bragg Healthy Way. Here's Prevention and Health Maintaince help all in one book.

I have my life back after years of chronic fatigue, fibromyalgia & clinical depression. I give thanks to Bragg Health Books.

– Marilyn Mason

0-87790-094-9 – $8.95

SUPER POWER BREATHING
FOR SUPER ENERGY
HIGH HEALTH & LONGEVITY

Breathing deeply, fully and completely energizes, calms, fills you with peace and keeps you youthful. Learn Bragg Breathing Exercises for more go-power and Super Health!

Thanks to Paul Bragg and Bragg Books, my years of asthma were cured in only one month with The Bragg Super Breathing and Bragg Healthy Lifestyle living!

0–87790–020–5 – $8.95   **– Paul Wenner**
Gardenburger Creator

"I thank Paul Bragg and the Bragg Healthy Lifestyle for my healthy, long, active life." I love Bragg Books and Health Products."
– Jack LaLanne, 90 years young, Bragg follower since 15

I have followed"The Bragg Healthy Lifestyle for years and it teaches you to take control of your health and build a healthy future."
– Mark Victor Hansen, Co-Author *Chicken Soup for thee Soul* Series

"Thanks to Bragg Books for my conversion to the healthy way."
– James F. Balch, M.D.
Co Author of – Prescription for Nutritional Healing

"Bragg Books have been a blessing to our family and the TBN family of loyal viewers"
– Evangelist Dwight Thompson
Co Host TBN "Praise The Lord"

If Bragg Books are unavailable in your area order:
On-line at: www.bragg.com or see booklist on back pages this book

154

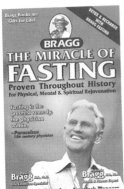
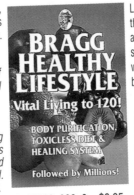
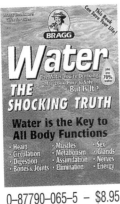
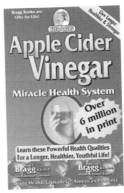
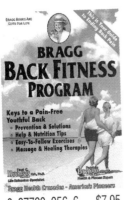
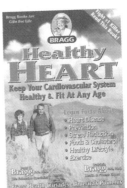

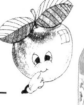

Send for Free Health Bulletins

Patricia Bragg wants to keep in touch with you, your relatives and friends about the latest Health, Nutrition, Exercise and Longevity Discoveries. Please enclose one stamp for each USA name listed. Foreign listings send postal reply coupons.

With Blessings of Health, Peace and Thanks,

Patricia

Please make copy, then print clearly and mail to:

BRAGG HEALTH CRUSADES, Box 7, Santa Barbara, CA 93102
You can help too!
Keep the Bragg Health Crusades "Crusading" with your tax-deductible gifts.

Name

Address   Apt. No.

City   State   Zip

Phone (   )   E-mail

Name

Address   Apt. No.

City   State   Zip

Phone (   )   E-mail

Name

Address   Apt. No.

City   State   Zip

Phone (   )   E-mail

Name

Address   Apt. No.

City   State   Zip

Phone (   )   E-mail

Name

Address   Apt. No.

City   State   Zip

Phone (   )   E-mail

Bragg Health Crusades spreading health worldwide since 1912

BRAGG ORGANIC APPLE CIDER VINEGAR

SIZE	PRICE	UPS SHIPPING & HANDLING For USA		$ Amount
16 oz.	$ 2.39 each	S/H – Please add $6 for 1st bottle and $1.50 each additional bottle		•
16 oz.	$23.00 Special Case /12	S/H Cost by Time Zone: CA $8. PST/MST $11. CST $15. EST $17.		•
32 oz.	$ 3.89 each	S/H – Please add $6 for 1st bottle and $2.00 each additional bottle		•
32 oz.	$41.00 Special Case /12	S/H Cost by Time Zone: CA $13. PST/MST $17. CST $24. EST $28.		•
1 gal.	$ 12.98 each	S/H 1st Bottle: CA $6. PST/MST $8. CST $9. EST $10. + $6 ea add. bottle		•
1 gal.	$ 47.00 Special Case /4	S/H Cost by Time Zone: CA $12. PST/MST $16. CST $23. EST $27.		•

Bragg Vinegar is a food and not taxable

Bragg VINEGAR	$	•
Shipping & Handling		•
TOTAL	$	•

BRAGG LIQUID AMINOS

SIZE	PRICE	UPS SHIPPING & HANDLING For USA		$ Amount
6 oz.	$ 2.98 each	S/H – Please add $4.00 for 1st 3 bottles – $1.25 each additional bottle		•
6 oz.	$ 65.00 Special Case /24	S/H Cost by Time Zone: CA $8. PST/MST $9. CST $11. EST $13.		•
16 oz.	$ 3.95 each	S/H – Please add $6 for 1st bottle – $1.25 each additional bottle		•
16 oz.	$42.00 Special Case /12	S/H Cost by Time Zone: CA $8. PST/MST $9. CST $13. EST $14.		•
32 oz.	$ 6.45 each	S/H – Please add $6 for 1st bottle – $2.00 each additional bottle		•
32 oz.	$70.00 Special Case /12	S/H Cost by Time Zone: CA $11. PST/MST $14. CST $21. EST $27.		•
1 gal.	$ 23.50 each	S/H 1st Bottle: CA $6. PST/MST $8. CST $9. EST $10. + $6 ea add. bottle		•
1 gal.	$ 79.00 Special Case /4	S/H Cost by Time Zone: CA $14. PST/MST $20. CST $25. EST $30.		•

Bragg Aminos is a food and not taxable

Bragg AMINOS	$	•
Shipping & Handling		•
TOTAL	$	•

BRAGG ORGANIC OLIVE OIL

SIZE	PRICE	USA SHIPPING & HANDLING		$ Amount
16 oz.	$ 8.95 each	S/H – Please add $6 for 1st bottle and $1.50 each additional bottle.		•
16 oz.	$ 95.00 Special Case /12	S/H Cost by Time Zone: CA $8. PST/MST $11. CST $15. EST $17.		•
32 oz.	$14.95 each	S/H – Please add $6 for 1st bottle and $2.00 each additional bottle		•
32 oz.	$149.50 Special Case /12	S/H Cost by Time Zone: CA $13. PST/MST $17. CST $24. EST $28.		•
1 gal.	$ 49.95 each	S/H Cost by Time Zone: CA $6. PST/MST $8. CST $9 EST $10. + $6 ea add. Btl.		•
1 gal.	$169.00 Special Case /4	S/H Cost by Time Zone: CA $12. PST/MST $16. CST $23. EST $27.		•

Bragg Olive Oil is a food and not taxable
Foreign orders, please inquire on postage

Please Specify: ☐ Check ☐ Money Order ☐ Cash
Charge To: ☐ Visa ☐ MasterCard ☐ Discover

Credit Card
Number: _____

Signature: _____

Bragg OLIVE OIL	$	•
Shipping & Handling		•
TOTAL	$	•

Card Expires: ____ / ____
month / year

Business office calls (805) 968-1020. We accept MasterCard, Discover & VISA phone orders. Please prepare order using order form. It speeds your call and serves as order record. Hours: 8 to 4 pm Pacific Time, Monday thru Thursday Visit our Web: www.bragg.com • e-mail: bragg@bragg.com

CREDIT CARD ORDERS
CALL (800) 446-1990 ☎
OR FAX (805) 968-1001

Mail to: **HEALTH SCIENCE, Box 7, Santa Barbara, CA 93102 USA**
Please Print or Type – Be sure to give street & house number to facilitate delivery.

Name _____

Address _____ Apt. No. _____

City _____ State _____ Zip _____

( ) _____
Phone   E-mail

Bragg Products are available at most Health Stores.

BOF 904

BRAGG "HOW-TO, SELF-HEALTH" BOOKS

Authored by America's First Family of Health
Live Longer – Healthier – Stronger Self-Improvement Library

Qty.	Bragg Book Titles ORDER FORM Health Science ISBN 0-87790	Price	$ Total
_____	**Get Healthy, Live Longer – 9 Book Offer** (Vegetarian Recipes / not Incl.) ...	69.00	•
_____	**Apple Cider Vinegar – Miracle Health System**	7.95	•
_____	**Bragg Healthy Lifestyle** – Vital Living to 120..............................	8.95	•
_____	**Miracle of Fasting** – Bragg Bible of Health for physical rejuvenation	9.95	•
_____	**Healthy Heart & Cardiovascular System** – Have fit heart at any age ...	8.95	•
_____	**Bragg Back Fitness Program for Pain-Free Strong Back**....................	7.95	•
_____	**Water – The Shocking Truth** That Can Save Your Life	8.95	•
_____	**Super Power Breathing** for Super Energy and High Health.................	8.95	•
_____	**Build Powerful Nerve Force** – reduce fatigue, stress, anger, anxiety	8.95	•
_____	**Build Strong Healthy Feet** – Dr. Scholl said it's the best	8.95	•
_____	**Bragg's Vegetarian Health Recipes** – Delicious & Nutritious	9.95	•

TOTAL COPIES Prices subject to change without notice.   **TOTAL BOOKS $**   •

CA Residents add sales tax   •

Please Specify: ☐ Check ☐ Money Order ☐ Cash

Shipping & Handling   •

(USA Funds Only)
TOTAL ENCLOSED $ •

Charge To: ☐ Visa ☐ Master Card ☐ Discover

Month   Year

VISA   _MasterCard_   _DISCOVER_

Card Expires

USA Shipping | Please add $4 first book $1 each additional book

USA retail book orders over $50 add $6 only

Foreign Shipping | Canada & Foreign orders add $5 first book, $1.50 @ additional book

Credit Card Number

Signature

Business office calls (805) 968-1020. We accept MasterCard, Discover or VISA phone orders. Please prepare order using this order form. It will speed your call and serve as your order record. Hours: 8 to 4 pm Pacific Time, Monday thru Thursday. **Visit our Web: www.bragg.com • e-mail: bragg@bragg.com**

CREDIT CARD ORDERS ONLY
CALL **(800) 446-1990**
OR FAX **(805) 968-1001**

See & Order Bragg 'Bound' Books, E-Books, & Products on www.bragg.com
Mail to: **HEALTH SCIENCE, Box 7, Santa Barbara, CA 93102 USA**

•
Name

•
Address   Apt. No.

•
City   State   Zip

Phone (   )   • E-mail   ˙BOF904

Bragg Books are available most Health & Book Stores – Nationwide

– Make copies when needed for mailing in. –

Send for Free Health Bulletins

Patricia Bragg wants to keep in touch with you, your relatives and friends about the latest Health, Nutrition, Exercise and Longevity Discoveries. Please enclose one stamp for each USA name listed. Foreign listings send postal reply coupons.

With Blessings of Health and Thanks, *Patricia*

Please make copy, then print clearly and mail to:

BRAGG HEALTH CRUSADES, Box 7, Santa Barbara, CA 93102

You can help too!

Keep the Bragg Health Crusades "Crusading" with your tax-deductible gifts.

Name

Address Apt. No.

City State Zip

Phone ( ) E-mail

Name

Address Apt. No.

City State Zip

Phone ( ) E-mail

Name

Address Apt. No.

City State Zip

Phone ( ) E-mail

Name

Address Apt. No.

City State Zip

Phone ( ) E-mail

Name

Address Apt. No.

City State Zip

Phone ( ) E-mail

Bragg Health Crusades spreading health worldwide since 1912

PAUL C. BRAGG, N.D., Ph.D.
Life Extension Specialist • World Health Crusader
Lecturer and Advisor to Olympic Athletes, Royalty and Stars
Originator of Health Food Stores – Now Worldwide

For almost a Century, Living Proof that his
"Health and Fitness Way of Life" Works Wonders!

Paul C. Bragg, Father of the Health Movement in America, had vision and dedication. This dynamic Crusader for worldwide health and fitness is responsible for more *firsts* in the history of the Health Movement than any other individual.

Bragg's amazing pioneering achievements the world now enjoys:

- Bragg originated, named and opened the first Health Food Store in America.
- Bragg Health Crusades pioneered the first Health Lectures across America. Bragg inspired followers to open Health Food Stores across America and also worldwide.
- Bragg was the first to introduce pineapple juice and tomato juice to America.
- He introduced Juice Therapy in America by importing the first hand-juicers.
- He was the first to introduce and distribute honey and date sugar nationwide.
- Bragg pioneered Radio Health Programs from Hollywood three times daily in the 20s.
- Bragg and daughter Patricia pioneered a Health TV show from Hollywood to spread The Bragg Health Crusade on their show, *Health and Happiness*. It included exercises, health recipes, visual demonstrations and guest appearances by famous, health-minded people.
- Bragg opened the first health restaurants and the first health spas in America.
- He created the first health foods and products and then made them available nationwide: herbal teas, health beverages, seven-grain cereals and crackers, health cosmetics, calcium, vitamins and mineral supplements, wheat germ, whey, digestive enzymes from papaya, sundried fruits, raw nuts, herbs and kelp seasonings, health candies, and amino acids from soybeans. Bragg inspired others to follow (Schiff, Gardenburger, Shaklee, TwinLabs, Trader Joe's, Herbalife, etc.) and now there are thousands of health items available worldwide!

Crippled by TB as a teenager, Bragg developed his own eating, breathing and exercising program to rebuild his body into an ageless, tireless, pain-free citadel of glowing, super health. He excelled in running, swimming, biking, progressive weight training and mountain climbing. He made an early pledge to God, in return for his renewed health, to spend the rest of his life showing others the road to super health. He honored his pledge! Paul Bragg's health pioneering made a difference worldwide.

A legend and beloved health crusader to millions, Bragg was the inspiration and personal health and fitness advisor to top Olympic Stars from 4-time swimming Gold Medalist Murray Rose to 3-time track Gold Medalist Betty Cuthbert of Australia, his relative (pole-vaulting Gold Medalist) Don Bragg, and countless others. Jack LaLanne, the original TV Fitness King , says, *"Bragg saved my life at age 15 when I attended the Bragg Crusade in Oakland, California."* From the earliest days, Bragg advised the greatest Hollywood Stars and giants of American Business, J C Penney, Del E. Webb, Dr. Scholl and Conrad Hilton are just a few who he inspired to long, successful, healthy, active lives!

Dr. Bragg changed the lives of millions worldwide in all walks of life with the Bragg Health Crusades, Books, Radio and TV appearances. (See and hear him on the web.)

BRAGG HEALTH CRUSADES, Box 7, SANTA BARBARA, CA 93102 USA • www.bragg.com

PATRICIA BRAGG, N.D., Ph.D.
Health Crusader & Angel of Health & Healing

Author, Lecturer, Nutritionist, Health Educator & Fitness Advisor to World Leaders, Hollywood Stars, Singers, Dancers, Athletes, etc.

Patricia is a 100% dedicated health crusader with a passion like her father, Paul C. Bragg, world renowned health authority. Patricia has won international fame on her own in this field. She conducts Health and Fitness Seminars for Women's, Men's, Youth and Church Groups throughout the world . . . and promotes Bragg "How-To, Self-Health" Books on Radio and Television Talk Shows throughout the English-speaking world. Consultants to Presidents and Royalty, to Stars of Stage, Screen and TV and to Champion Athletes, Patricia and her father co-authored The Bragg Health Library of Instructive, Inspiring Books that promote a healthier lifestyle, for a long, vital, happy life.

Patricia herself is the symbol of health, perpetual youth and radiant, feminine energy. She is a living and sparkling example of her and her father's healthy lifestyle precepts and this she loves sharing world-wide.

A fifth-generation Californian on her mother's side, Patricia was reared by The Bragg Natural Health Method from infancy. In school, she not only excelled in athletics, but also won honors for her studies and her counseling. She is an accomplished musician and dancer . . . as well as tennis player and mountain climber . . . and the youngest woman ever to be granted a U.S. Patent. Patricia is a popular gifted Health Teacher and a dynamic, in-demand Talk Show Guest where she spreads the simple, easy-to-follow Bragg Healthy Lifestyle for everyone of all ages.

Man's body is his vehicle through life, his earthly temple . . . and the Creator wants us filled with joy & health for a long fruitful life. The Bragg Crusades of Health and Fitness (3 John 2) has carried her around the world over 13 times – spreading physical, spiritual, emotional and mental health and joy. Health is our birthright and Patricia teaches how to prevent the destruction of our health from man-made wrong habits of living.

Patricia's been a Health Consultant to American Presidents and British Royalty, to Betty Cuthbert, Australia's "Golden Girl," who holds 16 world records and four Olympic gold medals in women's track and to New Zealand's Olympic Track and Triathlete Star, Allison Roe. Among those who come to her for advice are some of Hollywood's top Stars from Clint Eastwood to the ever-youthful singing group, The Beach Boys and their families, Singing Stars of the Metropolitan Opera and top Ballet Stars. Patricia's message is of world-wide appeal to people of all ages, nationalities and walks-of-life. Those who follow The Bragg Healthy Lifestyle and attend the Bragg Crusades world-wide are living testimonials . . . like ageless, super athlete, Jack LaLanne, who at age 15 went from sickness to Total Health!

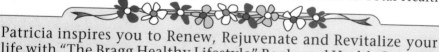

Patricia inspires you to Renew, Rejuvenate and Revitalize your life with "The Bragg Healthy Lifestyle" Books and Health Crusades worldwide. Millions have benefitted from these life-changing events with a longer, healthier and happier life! She loves to share with your community, organization, church groups, etc. Also, she is a perfect radio and TV talk show guest to spread the message of healthy lifestyle living. See and hear Patricia on the web: bragg.com

For Radio interview requests and info write or call (805) 968-1020
BRAGG HEALTH CRUSADES, BOX 7, SANTA BARBARA, CA 93102, USA